**General Surgery Residency Match Selection
Criteria and Programs Requirements.**

By

**Match A Doc
and
Residency Guide**

Table of Contents

Introduction

General Surgery Residency Match Criteria

Including the IMG Friendly General Surgery Residency Programs

This book is the must-read book and most single important piece you buy in your battle for residency. This is the General Surgery Residency Match Selection Criteria and Programs Requirements book that contains up-to-date information about all the programs in the United States for both AMGs and IMGs. Why this book is essential to match? It has been shown that applying to programs that you don't match their minimum criteria is just waste of money and time. It is very important that you apply to those programs that you meet their requirements and this why we decided to make your life easier by gathering the information you need in one book. The information was gathered from program directors, coordinators, chiefs, faculty and residents. It includes Programs names, Programs codes, States, Addresses, Phones,

Faxes, Percentage of IMGs in the programs, Minimum USMLE Step 1 and Step 2 Score Requirements, Attempts on any step, CS requirement at time of application, USCE Requirements, Cut-Off time since graduation, Programs offering couple match and Visas Sponsored or accepted. We have more than 10 years experience in the match field and our book is the proof that will help you to get the highest number of interviews to increase your chances in the match journey.

information here on your own
responsibility.

Alabama

Baptist Health System General Surgery Residency Program

Specialty: General Surgery
Program name: Baptist Health System Program
Program code: 440-01-21-020
NRMP Code: 1903440C0, 1903440P0
Program type: Community-based
State: Alabama
Address: Princeton Baptist Medical Center, POB III Suite 200,
          833 Princeton Ave SW, Birmingham,
AL 35211
Phone: (205) 783-3098
Fax: (205) 783-3164
Percentage of IMGs in the program: 10%

Minimum USMLE Step 1 Score Requirement: 205
Minimum USMLE Step 2 Score Requirement: 205
Attempts on any step: Must pass on first attempt including CS exam
CS required at time of application: Yes
USCE Requirement: None
Cut-Off time since graduation: No limits set
Program offers couple match: Yes
Visas Sponsored or accepted: J1 visa

University of Alabama Medical Center General Surgery Residency Program

Specialty: General Surgery
Program name: University of Alabama Medical Center Program
Program code: 440-01-21-022
NRMP Code: 1007440C0
Program type: University-based
State: Alabama
Address: University of Alabama Medical Center, Suite 321,
    1922 7th Ave S, Birmingham, AL 35294
Phone: (205) 934-9600 - (205) 996-7969
Percentage of IMGs in the program: 0%

Minimum USMLE Step 1 Score Requirement: No limits set
Minimum USMLE Step 2 Score Requirement: No limits set
Attempts on any step: Must pass on first attempt including CS exam
CS required at time of application: No
USCE Requirement: Yes
Cut-Off time since graduation: 7 years
Program offers couple match: Yes
Visas Sponsored or accepted: J1 visa and H1b visa

University of South Alabama General Surgery Residency Program

Specialty: General Surgery
Program name: University of South Alabama Program
Program code: 440-01-11-024
NRMP Code: 1852440C0
Program type: University-based
State: Alabama
Address: University of South Alabama Medical Center, Mastin 711,
        2451 Fillingim St, Mobile, AL 36617
Phone: (251) 471-7992
Fax: (251) 471-7022
Percentage of IMGs in the program: 15%

Minimum USMLE Step 1 Score Requirement: 205

Minimum USMLE Step 2 Score Requirement: 205

Attempts on any step: Must pass on first attempt

CS required at time of application: Yes including ECFMG certificate

USCE Requirement: None

Cut-Off time since graduation: No limits set

Program offers couple match: Yes

Visas Sponsored or accepted: No visa

Arizona

Banner Good Samaritan Medical Center General Surgery Program

Specialty: General Surgery

Program name: Banner Good Samaritan Medical Center Program

Program code: 440-03-22-026

NRMP Code: 1011440P1, 1011440C0

Program type: Community-based university affiliated hospital

State: Arizona

Address: Banner Good Samaritan Medical Center, 2nd Floor,
925 E McDowell Rd, Phoenix, AZ 85006
Phone: (602) 839-3339
Fax: (602) 839-3300
Percentage of IMGs in the program: 9%
Minimum USMLE Step 1 Score Requirement: 205
Minimum USMLE Step 2 Score Requirement: 205
Attempts on any step: No limits set
CS required at time of application: No
USCE Requirement: Yes
Cut-Off time since graduation: 3 years
Program offers couple match: Yes
Visas Sponsored or accepted: J1 visa

Maricopa Medical Center General Surgery Residency Program

Specialty: General Surgery
Program name: Maricopa Medical Center Program
Program code: 440-03-22-025
NRMP Code: 1898440C0, 1898440P0, 1898440P1
Program type: Community-based university affiliated hospital
State: Arizona

Address: Maricopa Medical Center, Department of Surgery,

        2601 E Roosevelt St, Phoenix, AZ 85008

Phone: (602) 344-5445
Fax: (602) 344-5048
Percentage of IMGs in the program: 15%
Minimum USMLE Step 1 Score Requirement: No limits set
Minimum USMLE Step 2 Score Requirement: No limits set
Attempts on any step: No limits set
CS required at time of application: No
USCE Requirement: None
Cut-Off time since graduation: No limits set
Program offers couple match: Yes
Visas Sponsored or accepted: No visa

College of Medicine Mayo Clinic (Arizona) General Surgery Residency Program

Specialty: General Surgery
Program name: Mayo Clinic College of Medicine (Arizona) Program
Program code: 440-03-21-402
NRMP Code: 3200440P0, 3200440C0
Program type: Community-based university affiliated hospital
State: Arizona

Address: Mayo Clinic Hospital, Department of Surgery,

        5779 E Mayo Blvd, Phoenix, AZ 85054

Phone: (480) 342-3093

Fax: (480) 342-2170

Percentage of IMGs in the program: 20%

Minimum USMLE Step 1 Score Requirement: 225

Minimum USMLE Step 2 Score Requirement: 225

Attempts on any step: Must pass on first attempt including CS attempt

CS required at time of application: No

USCE Requirement: None

Cut-Off time since graduation: 5 years

Program offers couple match: Yes

Visas Sponsored or accepted: J1 visa and H1b visa

College of Medicine Mayo Clinic (Arizona) General Surgery Residency Program

Specialty: General Surgery

Program name: Mayo Clinic College of Medicine (Arizona) Program

Program code: 440-03-21-402

NRMP Code: 3200440P0, 3200440C0

Program type: Community-based university affiliated hospital

State: Arizona
Address: Mayo Clinic Hospital, Department of Surgery,
             5779 E Mayo Blvd, Phoenix, AZ 85054
Phone: (480) 342-3093
Fax: (480) 342-2170
Percentage of IMGs in the program: 20%
Minimum USMLE Step 1 Score Requirement: 225
Minimum USMLE Step 2 Score Requirement: 225
Attempts on any step: Must pass on first attempt including CS attempt
CS required at time of application: No
USCE Requirement: None
Cut-Off time since graduation: 5 years
Program offers couple match: Yes
Visas Sponsored or accepted: J1 visa and H1b visa

University of Arizona General Surgery Residency Program

Specialty: General Surgery
Program name: University of Arizona Program
Program code: 440-03-21-027
NRMP Code: 1015440C0, 1015440P0, 1015440P1
Program type: University-based
State: Arizona

Address: University of Arizona Health Sciences Center, PO Box 245058,
1501 N Campbell Ave, Tucson, AZ 85724-5058
Phone: (520) 626-7747
Fax: (520) 626-2247
Percentage of IMGs in the program: 35%
Minimum USMLE Step 1 Score Requirement: 220
Minimum USMLE Step 2 Score Requirement: 220
Attempts on any step: No limits set
CS required at time of application: No
USCE Requirement: None
Cut-Off time since graduation: 5 years
Program offers couple match: Yes
Visas Sponsored or accepted: J1 visa

St. Joseph Hospital and Medical Center General Surgery Residency Program

Specialty: General Surgery
Program name: St Joseph's Hospital and Medical Center Program
Program code: 440-03-12-420
NRMP Code: 1012440C0, 1012440P0
Program type: Community-based university affiliated hospital
State: Arizona

Address: St Joseph's Hospital and Medical Center, Surgical Education,
      350 W Thomas Rd, Phoenix, AZ 85013
Phone: (602) 406-6540
Fax: (602) 406-4113
Percentage of IMGs in the program: 8%
Minimum USMLE Step 1 Score Requirement: No limits set
Minimum USMLE Step 2 Score Requirement: No limits set
Attempts on any step: No limits set
CS required at time of application: Yes including ECFMG certificate
USCE Requirement: None
Cut-Off time since graduation: 4 years
Program offers couple match: Yes
Visas Sponsored or accepted: J1 visa

Arkansas

University of Arkansas for Medical Sciences General Surgery Residency Program

Specialty: General Surgery
Program name: University of Arkansas for Medical Sciences Program

Program code: 440-04-21-029
NRMP Code: 1018440P0, 1018440C0
Program type: University-based
State: Arkansas
Address: University of Arkansas for Med Sciences, #520,
4301 W Markham St, Little Rock, AR 72205
Phone: (501) 686-6627
Fax: (501) 686-5696
Percentage of IMGs in the program: 0%
Minimum USMLE Step 1 Score Requirement: 230
Minimum USMLE Step 2 Score Requirement: 230
Attempts on any step: Must pass on first attempt including CS exam
CS required at time of application: No
USCE Requirement: No
Cut-Off time since graduation: No limits set
Program offers couple match: Yes
Visas Sponsored or accepted: J1 visa and H1b visa

California

Kaweah Delta Health Care District (KDHCD) General Surgery Residency Program

Specialty: General Surgery
Program name: Kaweah Delta Health Care District (KDHCD) Program
Program code: 440-05-00-428
State: California
Address: Kaweah Delta Health Care District
400 W Mineral King Ave, Visalia, CA 93291
Phone: (559) 624-5220
Fax: (559) 625-7680
Percentage of IMGs in the program: New program
Minimum USMLE Step 1 Score Requirement: No limits set
Minimum USMLE Step 2 Score Requirement: No limits set
Attempts on any step: Must pass maximum from 2nd attempt
CS required at time of application: No but PTAL/Status letter required
USCE Requirement: Yes
Cut-Off time since graduation: 5 years
Program offers couple match: Yes
Visas Sponsored or accepted: No visa

Cedars-Sinai Medical Center General Surgery Residency Program

Specialty: General Surgery
Program name: Cedars-Sinai Medical Center Program
Program code: 440-05-11-037
State: California
Address: Cedars-Sinai Medical Center
Department of Surgery, Suite 8215
8700 Beverly Blvd, Los Angeles, CA 90048
Phone: (310) 423-6637
Fax: (310) 388-0208
Percentage of IMGs in the program: 5%
Minimum USMLE Step 1 Score Requirement: 220
Minimum USMLE Step 2 Score Requirement: 220
Attempts on any step: Must pass on first attempt
CS required at time of application: Yes including ECFMG certificate and PTAL/Status letter
USCE Requirement: None
Cut-Off time since graduation: No limits set
Program offers couple match: Yes
Visas Sponsored or accepted: J1 visa

University of Southern California/LAC+USC Medical Center General Surgery Residency Program

Specialty: General Surgery
Program name: University of Southern California/LAC+USC Medical Center Program
Program code: 440-05-11-039
NRMP Code: 1033440C0, 1033440P3, 1033440P4
Program type: Community-based university affiliated hospital
State: California
Address: LAC+USC Medical Center
1520 San Pablo St, Los Angeles, CA 90033
Phone: (323) 442-5876
Fax: (323) 442-6887
Percentage of IMGs in the program: 20%
Minimum USMLE Step 1 Score Requirement: 220
Minimum USMLE Step 2 Score Requirement: 220
Attempts on any step: No limits set
CS required at time of application: Yes including ECFMG certificate and PTAL/Status letter
USCE Requirement: None
Cut-Off time since graduation: 5 years

Program offers couple match: Yes
Visas Sponsored or accepted: J1 visa

Huntington Memorial Hospital General Surgery Residency Program

Specialty: General Surgery
Program name: Huntington Memorial Hospital Program
Program code: 440-05-11-047
NRMP Code: 1044440P0, 1044440C0
Program type: Community-based university affiliated hospital
State: California
Address: Huntington Memorial Hospital
100 W California Blvd, Pasadena, CA 91105
Phone: (626) 397-5187
Fax: (626) 397-2914
Percentage of IMGs in the program: 0%
Minimum USMLE Step 1 Score Requirement: 210
Minimum USMLE Step 2 Score Requirement: 210
Attempts on any step: Must pass from first attempt
CS required at time of application: No
but PTAL/Status letter required
USCE Requirement: None

Cut-Off time since graduation: 5 years
Program offers couple match: No
Visas Sponsored or accepted: J1 visa and H1b visa

Kaiser Permanente Southern California (Los Angeles) General Surgery Residency Program

Specialty: General Surgery
Program name: Kaiser Permanente Southern California (Los Angeles) Program
Program code: 440-05-12-038
State: California
Address: Kaiser Permanente Los Angeles Medical Center
            4760 Sunset Blvd, Los Angeles, CA 90027
Phone: (323) 783-1431
Fax: (323) 783-8747
Percentage of IMGs in the program: 0%
Minimum USMLE Step 1 Score Requirement: 215
Minimum USMLE Step 2 Score Requirement: 215
Attempts on any step: Must pass on first attempt
CS required at time of application: Yes including ECFMG certificate and PTAL/Status letter

USCE Requirement: None
Cut-Off time since graduation: 2 years
Program offers couple match: Yes
Visas Sponsored or accepted: H1b visa

Santa Barbara Cottage Hospital General Surgery Residency Program

Specialty: General Surgery
Program name: Santa Barbara Cottage Hospital Program
Program code: 440-05-12-053
State: California
Address: Santa Barbara Cottage Hospital
400 W Pueblo St, Santa Barbara, CA 93105
Phone: (805) 569-7316
Fax: (805) 569-7317
Percentage of IMGs in the program: 20%
Minimum USMLE Step 1 Score Requirement: 220
Minimum USMLE Step 2 Score Requirement: 220
Attempts on any step: No limits set
CS required at time of application: Yes including ECFMG certificate and PTAL/Status letter
USCE Requirement: Yes
Cut-Off time since graduation: No limits set

Program offers couple match: Yes
Visas Sponsored or accepted: No visa

San Joaquin General Hospital General Surgery Residency Program

Specialty: General Surgery
Program name: San Joaquin General Hospital Program
Program code: 440-05-12-055
State: California
Address: San Joaquin General Hospital
500 W Hospital Rd, French Camp, CA 95231-1020
Phone: (209) 468-6620
Fax: (209) 468-6246
Percentage of IMGs in the program: 25%
Minimum USMLE Step 1 Score Requirement: 220
Minimum USMLE Step 2 Score Requirement: 220
Attempts on any step: Must pass on first attempt including CS exam
CS required at time of application: Yes including ECFMG certificate and PTAL/Status letter
USCE Requirement: None
Cut-Off time since graduation: 2 years
Program offers couple match: No

Visas Sponsored or accepted: J1 visa

University of California (Davis) Health System General Surgery Residency Program

Specialty: General Surgery
Program name: University of California (Davis) Health System Program
Program code: 440-05-21-031
NRMP Code: 1046440P0, 1046440C0
Program type: University-based
State: California
Address: UC Davis Medical Center
2315 Stockton Blvd, Sacramento, CA 95817-2282
Phone: (916) 734-2724
Fax: (916) 734-5633
Percentage of IMGs in the program: 0%
Minimum USMLE Step 1 Score Requirement: 220
Minimum USMLE Step 2 Score Requirement: 220
Attempts on any step: No limits set
CS required at time of application: Yes including ECFMG certificate and PTAL/Status letter
USCE Requirement: None
Cut-Off time since graduation: No limits set
Program offers couple match: Yes

Visas Sponsored or accepted: J1 visa

University of California (San Francisco)/Fresno General Surgery Residency Program

Specialty: General Surgery
Program name: University of California (San Francisco)/Fresno Program
Program code: 440-05-21-032
NRMP Code: 1022440C0
Program type: Community-based university affiliated hospital
State: California
Address: UCSF Fresno
          155 N Fresno St, Fresno, CA 93701
Phone: (559) 459-5196
Fax: (559) 459-3719
Percentage of IMGs in the program: 0%
Minimum USMLE Step 1 Score Requirement: 225
Minimum USMLE Step 2 Score Requirement: 225
Attempts on any step: No limits set
CS required at time of application: Yes including ECFMG certificate and PTAL/Status letter
USCE Requirement: None
Cut-Off time since graduation: No limits set
Program offers couple match: Yes

Visas Sponsored or accepted: J1 visa

University of California (Irvine) General Surgery Residency Program

Specialty: General Surgery
Program name: University of California (Irvine) Program
Program code: 440-05-21-033
NRMP Code: 1043440C0, 1043440P0, 1043440P1
Program type: University-based
State: California
Address: UC Irvine Medical Center
            333 City Blvd W, Orange, CA 92868
Phone: (714) 456-5532
Fax: (714) 456-7207
Percentage of IMGs in the program: 7%
Minimum USMLE Step 1 Score Requirement: No limits set
Minimum USMLE Step 2 Score Requirement: No limits set
Attempts on any step: No limits set
CS required at time of application: Yes including ECFMG certificate and PTAL/Status letter
USCE Requirement: None
Cut-Off time since graduation: No limits set
Program offers couple match: Yes

Visas Sponsored or accepted: J1 visa

Loma Linda University General Surgery Residency Program

Specialty: General Surgery
Program name: Loma Linda University Program
Program code: 440-05-21-034
State: California
Address: Loma Linda University Medical Center
11175 Campus St, Loma Linda, CA 92354
Phone: (909) 558-4289
Fax: (909) 558-4872
Percentage of IMGs in the program: 10%
Minimum USMLE Step 1 Score Requirement: 210
Minimum USMLE Step 2 Score Requirement: 210
Attempts on any step: Must pass on first attempt including CS exam
CS required at time of application: Yes including ECFMG certificate and PTAL/Status letter
USCE Requirement: None
Cut-Off time since graduation: No limits set
Program offers couple match: Yes
Visas Sponsored or accepted: J1 visa and H1b visa

UCLA Medical Center General Surgery General Surgery Residency Program

Specialty: General Surgery
Program name: UCLA Medical Center Program
Program code: 440-05-21-042
NRMP Code: 1956440C0, 1956440P2, 1956440P0
Program type: University-based
State: California
Address: David Geffen School of Medicine UCLA 10833 Le Conte Ave, Los Angeles, CA 90095-1749
Phone: (310) 206-9291
Fax: (310) 267-0369
Percentage of IMGs in the program: 5%
Minimum USMLE Step 1 Score Requirement: 225
Minimum USMLE Step 2 Score Requirement: 225
Attempts on any step: Must pass on first attempt
CS required at time of application: No but PTAL/Status letter is required
USCE Requirement: None
Cut-Off time since graduation: No limits set
Program offers couple match: Yes
Visas Sponsored or accepted: J1 visa

University of California (San Diego) General Surgery Residency Program

Specialty: General Surgery
Program name: University of California (San Diego) Program
Program code: 440-05-21-048
State: California
Address: UCSD Medical Center
200 W Arbor Dr, San Diego, CA 92103
Phone: (619) 471-3859
Fax: (619) 543-3017
Percentage of IMGs in the program: 0%
Minimum USMLE Step 1 Score Requirement: No limits set
Minimum USMLE Step 2 Score Requirement: No limits set
Attempts on any step: No limits set
CS required at time of application: No but PTAL/Status letter is required
USCE Requirement: None
Cut-Off time since graduation: No limits set
Program offers couple match: Yes
Visas Sponsored or accepted: No visa

University of California (San Francisco) General Surgery Residency Program

Specialty: General Surgery
Program name: University of California (San Francisco) Program
Program code: 440-05-21-052
State: California
Address: UCSF Medical Center
513 Parnassus Ave, San Francisco, CA 94143-0470
Phone: (415) 476-1239
Fax: (415) 502-1259
Percentage of IMGs in the program: 0%
Minimum USMLE Step 1 Score Requirement: No limits set
Minimum USMLE Step 2 Score Requirement: No limits set
Attempts on any step: No limits set
CS required at time of application: Yes including ECFMG certificate and PTAL/Status letter
USCE Requirement: None
Cut-Off time since graduation: No limits set
Program offers couple match: Yes
Visas Sponsored or accepted: J1 visa

Stanford University General Surgery Residency Program

Specialty: General Surgery
Program name: Stanford University Program
Program code: 440-05-21-054
State: California
Address: Stanford University Medical Center
300 Pasteur Dr, Stanford, CA 94305-5641
Phone: (650) 725-2181
Fax: (650) 724-9806
Percentage of IMGs in the program: 0%
Minimum USMLE Step 1 Score Requirement: No limits set
Minimum USMLE Step 2 Score Requirement: No limits set
Attempts on any step: No limits set
CS required at time of application: No but PTAL/Status letter required
USCE Requirement: None
Cut-Off time since graduation: 2 years
Program offers couple match: Yes
Visas Sponsored or accepted: J1 visa

Los Angeles County-Harbor-UCLA Medical Center General Surgery Residency Program

Specialty: General Surgery
Program name: Los Angeles County-Harbor-UCLA Medical Center Program
Program code: 440-05-21-056
State: California
Address: Los Angeles County-Harbor-UCLA Medical Center
           1000 W Carson St, Torrance, CA 90502
Phone: (310) 222-2700
Fax: (310) 533-1841
Percentage of IMGs in the program: 0%
Minimum USMLE Step 1 Score Requirement: No limits set
Minimum USMLE Step 2 Score Requirement: No limits set
Attempts on any step: No limits set
CS required at time of application: No but PTAL/Status letter required
USCE Requirement: None
Cut-Off time since graduation: No limits set
Program offers couple match: Yes
Visas Sponsored or accepted: J1 visa

University of California San Francisco (East Bay) General Surgery Residency Program

Specialty: General Surgery
Program name: University of California San Francisco (East Bay) Program

Program code: 440-05-21-389
NRMP Code: 3625440C0, 3625440P0
Program type: Community-based university affiliated hospital
State: California
Address: UCSF Medical Center-East Bay
1411 E 31st St, Oakland, CA 94602
Phone: (510) 437-4965
Fax: (510) 437-5017
Percentage of IMGs in the program: 0%
Minimum USMLE Step 1 Score Requirement: 220
Minimum USMLE Step 2 Score Requirement: 220
Attempts on any step: No limits set
CS required at time of application: Yes including ECFMG certificate and PTAL/Status letter
USCE Requirement: None
Cut-Off time since graduation: No limits set
Program offers couple match: Yes
Visas Sponsored or accepted: J1 visa

Riverside County Regional Medical Center General Surgery Residency Program

Specialty: General Surgery
Program name: Riverside County Regional Medical Center Program

Program code: 440-05-21-427
State: California
Address: Riverside County Regional Medical Center
26520 Cactus Ave, Moreno Valley, CA 92555
Phone: (951) 486-4853
Fax: (951) 486-5910
Percentage of IMGs in the program: 0%
Minimum USMLE Step 1 Score Requirement: No limits set
Minimum USMLE Step 2 Score Requirement: No limits set
Attempts on any step: No limits set
CS required at time of application: Yes including ECFMG certificate and PTAL/Status letter
USCE Requirement: None
Cut-Off time since graduation: 5 years
Program offers couple match: Yes
Visas Sponsored or accepted: No visa

Kern Medical Center General Surgery Residency Program

Specialty: General Surgery
Program name: Kern Medical Center Program
Program code: 440-05-31-030
NRMP Code: 1921440C0, 1921440P0
Program type: Community-based university

affiliated hospital
State: California
Address: Kern Medical Center
        1700 Mount Vernon Ave, Bakersfield,
CA 93306
Phone: (661) 326-2276
Fax: (661) 326-2282
Percentage of IMGs in the program: 30%
Minimum USMLE Step 1 Score Requirement:
No limits set
Minimum USMLE Step 2 Score Requirement:
No limits set
Attempts on any step: No limits set
CS required at time of application: Yes
including ECFMG certificate and PTAL/Status
letter
USCE Requirement: None
Cut-Off time since graduation: 2 years
Program offers couple match: Yes
Visas Sponsored or accepted: No visa

Arrowhead Regional Medical Center/Kaiser Permanente (Fontana) Program

Specialty: General Surgery
Program name: Arrowhead Regional Medical
Center/Kaiser Permanente (Fontana) Program
Program code: 440-05-31-425
State: California

Address: Arrowhead Regional Medical Center/Kaiser

        9961 Sierra Ave, Fontana, CA 92335

Phone: (909) 427-5626

Fax: (909) 427-4065

Percentage of IMGs in the program: 0%

Minimum USMLE Step 1 Score Requirement: No limits set

Minimum USMLE Step 2 Score Requirement: No limits set

Attempts on any step: No limits set

CS required at time of application: Yes including ECFMG certificate and PTAL/Status letter

USCE Requirement: None

Cut-Off time since graduation: 5 years

Program offers couple match: Yes

Visas Sponsored or accepted: No visa

Colorado

Exempla St Joseph Hospital General Surgery Residency Program

Specialty: General Surgery

Program name: Exempla St Joseph Hospital Program
Program code: 440-07-22-057
State: Colorado
Address: Exempla St Joseph Hospital
1835 Franklin St, Denver, CO 80218
Phone: (303) 837-7295
Fax: (303) 866-8044
Percentage of IMGs in the program: 10%
Minimum USMLE Step 1 Score Requirement: 220
Minimum USMLE Step 2 Score Requirement: 220
Attempts on any step: Must pass on first attempt including CS exam
CS required at time of application: No
USCE Requirement: Yes, 12 months
Cut-Off time since graduation: 4 years
Program offers couple match: Yes
Visas Sponsored or accepted: No visa

University of Colorado Denver General Surgery Residency Program

Specialty: General Surgery
Program name: University of Colorado Denver Program
Program code: 440-07-21-058

NRMP Code: 1076440C0, 1076440P0, 1076440P1
Program type: University-based
State: Colorado
Address: University of Colorado Denver School of Medicine

      12631 E 17th Ave, Aurora, CO 80045
Phone: (303) 724-2680
Fax: (303) 724-2682
Percentage of IMGs in the program: 0%
Minimum USMLE Step 1 Score Requirement: No limits set
Minimum USMLE Step 2 Score Requirement: No limits set
Attempts on any step: No limits set
CS required at time of application: Yes including ECFMG certificate
USCE Requirement: None
Cut-Off time since graduation: No limits set
Program offers couple match: Yes
Visas Sponsored or accepted: J1 visa and H1b visa

Connecticut

St Mary's Hospital (Waterbury) General Surgery Residency Program

Specialty: General Surgery
Program name: St Mary's Hospital (Waterbury) Program
Program code: 440-08-31-065
State: Connecticut
Address: St Mary's Hospital
          56 Franklin St, Waterbury, CT 06706
Phone: (203) 709-6479
Fax: (203) 709-6089
Percentage of IMGs in the program: 100%
Minimum USMLE Step 1 Score Requirement: 220
Minimum USMLE Step 2 Score Requirement: 220
Attempts on any step: Must pass on first attempt including CS exam
CS required at time of application: No
USCE Requirement: None
Cut-Off time since graduation: 3 years
Program offers couple match: Yes
Visas Sponsored or accepted: J1 visa

University of Connecticut General Surgery Residency Program

Specialty: General Surgery
Program name: University of Connecticut Program
Program code: 440-08-21-390
NRMP Code: 1094440P1, 1094440C0, 1094440P0
Program type: University-based
State: Connecticut
Address: University of Connecticut Health Center
           263 Farmington Ave, Farmington, CT 06030-3955
Phone: (860) 679-3467
Fax: (860) 679-1276
Percentage of IMGs in the program: 30%
Minimum USMLE Step 1 Score Requirement: 220
Minimum USMLE Step 2 Score Requirement: 220
Attempts on any step: Must pass on first attempt including CS exam
CS required at time of application: Yes including ECFMG certificate
USCE Requirement: None
Cut-Off time since graduation: 8 years
Program offers couple match: Yes
Visas Sponsored or accepted: J1 visa

Stamford Hospital/Columbia University College of Physicians and Surgeons General Surgery Residency Program

Specialty: General Surgery
Program name: Stamford Hospital/Columbia University College of Physicians and Surgeons Program
Program code: 440-08-21-364
NRMP Code: 1095440P0, 1095440C0
Program type: Community-based university affiliated hospital
State: Connecticut
Address: Stamford Hospital
   30 Shelburne Rd, Stamford, CT 06904
Phone: (203) 276-7467
Fax: (203) 276-7020
Percentage of IMGs in the program: 30%
Minimum USMLE Step 1 Score Requirement: 210
Minimum USMLE Step 2 Score Requirement: 210
Attempts on any step: Must pass on first attempt
CS required at time of application: No
USCE Requirement: Yes
Cut-Off time since graduation: 2 years
Program offers couple match: Yes
Visas Sponsored or accepted: No visa

Yale-New Haven Medical Center General Surgery Residency Program

Specialty: General Surgery
Program name: Yale-New Haven Medical Center Program
Program code: 440-08-21-064
State: Connecticut
Address: Yale-New Haven Medical Center
330 Cedar St, New Haven, CT 06520-8062
Phone: (203) 785-7890
Fax: (203) 737-5209
Percentage of IMGs in the program: 25%
Minimum USMLE Step 1 Score Requirement: No limits set
Minimum USMLE Step 2 Score Requirement: No limits set
Attempts on any step: No limits set
CS required at time of application: No
USCE Requirement: None
Cut-Off time since graduation: No limits set
Program offers couple match: Yes
Visas Sponsored or accepted: J1 visa

Danbury Hospital General Surgery Residency Program

Specialty: General Surgery
Program name: Danbury Hospital Program
Program code: 440-08-13-428
NRMP Code: 1081440P0, 1081440C0
Program type: Community-based university affiliated hospital
State: Connecticut
Address: Danbury Hospital
        111 Osborne St, Danbury, CT 06810
Phone: (203) 739-7844
Fax: (203) 739-8657
Percentage of IMGs in the program: 60%
Minimum USMLE Step 1 Score Requirement: No limits set
Minimum USMLE Step 2 Score Requirement: No limits set
Attempts on any step: Must pass on first attempt
CS required at time of application: No
USCE Requirement: None
Cut-Off time since graduation: 10 years
Program offers couple match: No
Visas Sponsored or accepted: J1 visa and H1b visa

Waterbury Hospital Health Center General Surgery Residency Program

Specialty: General Surgery
Program name: Waterbury Hospital Health Center Program
Program code: 440-08-11-066
NRMP Code: 1097440P0, 1097440C0
Program type: Community-based university affiliated hospital
State: Connecticut
Address: Waterbury Hospital
64 Robbins St, Waterbury, CT 06708
Phone: (203) 573-7256
Fax: (203) 573-6073
Percentage of IMGs in the program: 90%
Minimum USMLE Step 1 Score Requirement: 200
Minimum USMLE Step 2 Score Requirement: 205
Attempts on any step: Must pass on first attempt including CS exam
CS required at time of application: Yes
USCE Requirement: 6 months
Cut-Off time since graduation: 5 years
Program offers couple match: No
Visas Sponsored or accepted: J1 visa

Delaware

Christiana Care Health Services General Surgery Residency Program

Specialty: General Surgery
Program name: Christiana Care Health Services Program
Program code: 440-09-11-067
NRMP Code: 1099440C0
Program type: Community-based university affiliated hospital
State: Delaware
Address: Christiana Care Health System
4755 Ogletown-Stanton Rd, Newark, DE 19718
Phone: (302) 733-4503
Fax: (302) 733-4513
Percentage of IMGs in the program: 10%
Minimum USMLE Step 1 Score Requirement: 200
Minimum USMLE Step 2 Score Requirement: 205
Attempts on any step: No limits set
CS required at time of application: Yes as well as ECFMG certificate
USCE Requirement: Yes

Cut-Off time since graduation: No limits set
Program offers couple match: Yes
Visas Sponsored or accepted: J1 visa

District of Columbia

Washington Hospital Center General Surgery Residency Program

Specialty: General Surgery
Program name: Washington Hospital Center Program
Program code: 440-10-31-071
State: District of Columbia
Address: Washington Hospital Center, Suite G-253,
110 Irving St NW, Washington, DC 20010
Phone: (202) 877-3536
Fax: (202) 877-3699
Percentage of IMGs in the program: 11%
Minimum USMLE Step 1 Score Requirement: 200
Minimum USMLE Step 2 Score Requirement: 205

Attempts on any step: Must pass on first attempt including CS exam
CS required at time of application: Yes including ECFMG certificate
USCE Requirement: None
Cut-Off time since graduation: No limits set
Program offers couple match: Yes
Visas Sponsored or accepted: J1 visa

Howard University General Surgery Residency Program

Specialty: General Surgery
Program name: Howard University Program
Program code: 440-10-21-070
Program type: University-based
State: District of Columbia
Address: Howard University Hospital, Department of Surgery Room 4-B17,
          2041 Georgia Ave NW, Washington, DC 20060
Phone: (202) 865-1446
Fax: (202) 865-6728
Percentage of IMGs in the program: 20%
Minimum USMLE Step 1 Score Requirement: No limits set
Minimum USMLE Step 2 Score Requirement: No limits set
Attempts on any step: No limits set
CS required at time of application: No

USCE Requirement: None
Cut-Off time since graduation: No limits set
Program offers couple match: No
Visas Sponsored or accepted: J1 visa and H1b visa

Georgetown University Hospital General Surgery Residency Program

Specialty: General Surgery
Program name: Georgetown University Hospital Program
Program code: 440-10-21-068
State: District of Columbia
Address: Georgetown University Hospital, Surgical Education 2 Gorman Room 2051,
3800 Reservoir Rd NW, Washington, DC 20007-2113
Phone: (202) 444-8893
Fax: (202) 444-7422
Percentage of IMGs in the program: 0%
Minimum USMLE Step 1 Score Requirement: 220
Minimum USMLE Step 2 Score Requirement: 220
Attempts on any step: No limits set
CS required at time of application: Yes as well as ECFMG certificate
USCE Requirement: None

Cut-Off time since graduation: 2 years
Program offers couple match: Yes
Visas Sponsored or accepted: J1 visa

George Washington University General Surgery Residency Program

Specialty: General Surgery
Program name: George Washington University Program
Program code: 440-10-21-069
Program type: University-based
State: District of Columbia
Address: George Washington University Medical Center,
Department of Surgery Suite 6B,
2150 Pennsylvania Ave NW,
Washington, DC 20037
Phone: (202) 741-3157
Fax: (202) 741-3285
Percentage of IMGs in the program: 25%
Minimum USMLE Step 1 Score Requirement: 230
Minimum USMLE Step 2 Score Requirement: 230
Attempts on any step: No limits set
CS required at time of application: Yes as well as ECFMG certificate

USCE Requirement: None
Cut-Off time since graduation: No limits set
Program offers couple match: Yes
Visas Sponsored or accepted: J1 visa

Florida

University of South Florida Morsani General Surgery Residency Program

Specialty: General Surgery
Program name: University of South Florida Morsani Program
Program code: 440-11-31-078
State: Florida
Address: USF Health Morsani College of Medicine
2 Tampa General Circle, Tampa, FL 33606
Phone: (813) 259-8510
Fax: (813) 259-8660
Percentage of IMGs in the program: 15%
Minimum USMLE Step 1 Score Requirement: 220

Minimum USMLE Step 2 Score Requirement: 220

Attempts on any step: Must pass on first attempt including CS exam

CS required at time of application: No

USCE Requirement: None

Cut-Off time since graduation: 5 years unless clinically active

Program offers couple match: No

Visas Sponsored or accepted: J1 visa

Mount Sinai Medical Center of Florida General Surgery Residency Program

Specialty: General Surgery

Program name: Mount Sinai Medical Center of Florida Program

Program code: 440-11-22-075

NRMP Code: 1105440C0, 1105440P0

Program type: Community-based university affiliated hospital

State: Florida

Address: Mount Sinai Medical Center Florida 4306 Alton Rd, Miami Beach, FL 33140

Phone: (305) 695-1255

Fax: (305) 674-2781

Percentage of IMGs in the program: 30%

Minimum USMLE Step 1 Score Requirement: 200
Minimum USMLE Step 2 Score Requirement: 205
Attempts on any step: Must pass on first attempt
CS required at time of application: No
USCE Requirement: None
Cut-Off time since graduation: 5 years
Program offers couple match: No
Visas Sponsored or accepted: J1 visa

University of Miami Miller School of Medicine/Palm Beach Regional Campus General Surgery Residency Program

Specialty: General Surgery
Program name: University of Miami Miller School of Medicine/Palm Beach Regional Campus Program
Program code: 440-11-21-431
NRMP Code: 1384440C0
Program type: Community-based university affiliated hospital
State: Florida
Address: JFK Medical Center
        5301 S Congress Ave, Atlantis, FL 33462
Phone: (561) 548-1711

Fax: (561) 548-1743
Percentage of IMGs in the program: 50%
Minimum USMLE Step 1 Score Requirement: 210
Minimum USMLE Step 2 Score Requirement: 210
Attempts on any step: No limits set
CS required at time of application: No
USCE Requirement: None
Cut-Off time since graduation: No limits set
Program offers couple match: Yes
Visas Sponsored or accepted: J1 visa

Mayo Clinic College of Medicine (Jacksonville) General Surgery Residency Program

Specialty: General Surgery
Program name: Mayo Clinic College of Medicine (Jacksonville) Program
Program code: 440-11-21-405
NRMP Code: 1032440C0, 1032440P1, 1032440P0
Program type: University-based
State: Florida
Address: Mayo Clinic Jacksonville
 4500 San Pablo Rd, Jacksonville, FL 32224
Phone: (904) 953-0424

Fax: (904) 953-0430
Percentage of IMGs in the program: 0%
Minimum USMLE Step 1 Score Requirement: 220
Minimum USMLE Step 2 Score Requirement: 220
Attempts on any step: Must pass on first attempt including CS exam
CS required at time of application: Yes including ECFMG certificate
USCE Requirement: None
Cut-Off time since graduation: No limits set
Program offers couple match: Yes
Visas Sponsored or accepted: J1 visa and H1b visa

Jackson Memorial Hospital/Jackson Health System General Surgery Residency Program

Specialty: General Surgery
Program name: Jackson Memorial Hospital/Jackson Health System Program
Program code: 440-11-21-074
State: Florida
Address: Jackson Memorial Medical Center
            PO Box 016310, Miami, FL 33101
Phone: (305) 585-1280
Fax: (305) 585-6043
Percentage of IMGs in the program: 20%

Minimum USMLE Step 1 Score Requirement: 210

Minimum USMLE Step 2 Score Requirement: 210

Attempts on any step: Must pass on first attempt

CS required at time of application: Yes

USCE Requirement: None

Cut-Off time since graduation: No limits set

Program offers couple match: Yes

Visas Sponsored or accepted: J1 visa

University of Florida College of Medicine Jacksonville General Surgery Residency Program

Specialty: General Surgery

Program name: University of Florida College of Medicine Jacksonville Program

Program code: 440-11-21-073

NRMP Code: 1101440P0, 1101440C0

Program type: University-based

State: Florida

Address: University of Florida College of Medicine Jacksonville

653 W 8th St, Jacksonville, FL 32209

Phone: (904) 244-3903

Fax: (904) 244-3020

Percentage of IMGs in the program: 50%

Minimum USMLE Step 1 Score Requirement: 210
Minimum USMLE Step 2 Score Requirement: 210
Attempts on any step: Must pass maximum on 2nd attempt including CS exam
CS required at time of application: No
USCE Requirement: None
Cut-Off time since graduation: No limits set
Program offers couple match: Yes
Visas Sponsored or accepted: J1 visa

University of Florida General Surgery Residency Program

Specialty: General Surgery
Program name: University of Florida Program
Program code: 440-11-21-072
NRMP Code: 1824440C0, 1824440P0
Program type: University-based
State: Florida
Address: University of Florida College of Medicine
PO Box 100287, Gainesville, FL 32610-0287
Phone: (352) 265-0916
Fax: (352) 265-3292
Percentage of IMGs in the program: 20%
Minimum USMLE Step 1 Score Requirement: 220

Minimum USMLE Step 2 Score Requirement: 220
Attempts on any step: Must pass on first attempt
CS required at time of application: No
USCE Requirement: None
Cut-Off time since graduation: 2 years
Program offers couple match: Yes
Visas Sponsored or accepted: J1 visa

Cleveland Clinic (Florida) General Surgery Residency Program

Specialty: General Surgery
Program name: Cleveland Clinic (Florida) Program
Program code: 440-11-13-432
NRMP Code: 1383440P0, 1383440C0
Program type: Community-based university affiliated hospital
State: Florida
Address: Cleveland Clinic Florida
          2950 Cleveland Clinic Blvd, Weston, FL 33331
Phone: (954) 659-5815
Fax: (954) 659-5622
Percentage of IMGs in the program: 40%
Minimum USMLE Step 1 Score Requirement: 210

Minimum USMLE Step 2 Score Requirement: 210
Attempts on any step: Must pass first attempt
CS required at time of application: Yes
USCE Requirement: None
Cut-Off time since graduation: No limits set
Program offers couple match: Yes
Visas Sponsored or accepted: J1 visa and H1b visa

Halifax Medical Center General Surgery Residency Program

Specialty: General Surgery
Program name: Halifax Medical Center Program
Program code: 440-11-12-434
NRMP Code: 1629440C0
Program type: Community-based university affiliated hospital
State: Florida
Address: Halifax Health Medical Center
201 N Clyde Morris Blvd, Daytona Beach, FL 32114
Phone: (386) 226-4537
Fax: (386) 254-4285
Percentage of IMGs in the program: 25%
Minimum USMLE Step 1 Score Requirement: 210
Minimum USMLE Step 2 Score Requirement: 210

Attempts on any step: No limits set
CS required at time of application: No
USCE Requirement: Yes, 12 months
Cut-Off time since graduation: 3 years
Program offers couple match: Yes
Visas Sponsored or accepted: No visa

Florida Hospital Medical Center General Surgery Residency Program

Specialty: General Surgery
Program name: Florida Hospital Medical Center Program
Program code: 440-11-12-416
NRMP Code: 1102440C0
Program type: Community-based university affiliated hospital
State: Florida
Address: Florida Hosp Medical Center
2501 N Orange Ave, Orlando, FL 32804
Phone: (407) 303-7203
Fax: (407) 303-2469
Percentage of IMGs in the program: 20%
Minimum USMLE Step 1 Score Requirement: 210
Minimum USMLE Step 2 Score Requirement: 215

Attempts on any step: Must pass from first attempt including CS exam
CS required at time of application: Yes including ECFMG certificate
USCE Requirement: Yes
Cut-Off time since graduation: 5 years
Program offers couple match: Yes
Visas Sponsored or accepted: J1 visa and H1b visa

Orlando Health General Surgery Residency Program

Specialty: General Surgery
Program name: Orlando Health Program
Program code: 440-11-11-076
NRMP Code: 1107440C0, 1107440P0
Program type: Community-based university affiliated hospital
State: Florida
Address: Orlando Regional Medical Center
          86 W Underwood St, Orlando, FL 32806
Phone: (407) 841-5142
Fax: (407) 648-3686
Percentage of IMGs in the program: 0%
Minimum USMLE Step 1 Score Requirement: No limits set
Minimum USMLE Step 2 Score Requirement: No limits set

Attempts on any step: No limits set
CS required at time of application: No
USCE Requirement: None
Cut-Off time since graduation: 2 years
Program offers couple match: Yes
Visas Sponsored or accepted: No visa

Kendall Regional Medical Center General Surgery Residency Program

Specialty: General Surgery
Program name: Kendall Regional Medical Center Program
Program code: 440-11-00-435
State: Florida
Address: Kendall Regional Medical Center
11760 Bird Rd, Miami, FL 33175
Phone: (786) 315-5935
Fax: (305) 227-5556
Percentage of IMGs in the program: New program
Minimum USMLE Step 1 Score Requirement: 205
Minimum USMLE Step 2 Score Requirement: 210
Attempts on any step: Must pass on first attempt
CS required at time of application: No
USCE Requirement: None

Cut-Off time since graduation: 5 years
Program offers couple match: Yes
Visas Sponsored or accepted: No visa

Georgia

Memorial Health-University Medical Center/Mercer University School of Medicine (Savannah) General Surgery Residency Program

Specialty: General Surgery
Program name: Memorial Health-University Medical Center/Mercer University School of Medicine (Savannah) Program
Program code: 440-12-31-084
NRMP Code: 1971440C0
Program type: University-based
State: Georgia
Address: Memorial University Medical Center
4700 Waters Ave, Savannah, GA 31404
Phone: (912) 350-8598
Fax: (912) 350-5984
Percentage of IMGs in the program: 0%

Minimum USMLE Step 1 Score Requirement: No limits set

Minimum USMLE Step 2 Score Requirement: No limits set

Attempts on any step: Must pass on first attempt except for CS exam you are allowed to pass on the 2nd attempt

CS required at time of application: Yes

USCE Requirement: None

Cut-Off time since graduation: 2 years

Program offers couple match: Yes

Visas Sponsored or accepted: No visa

Medical College of Georgia General Surgery Residency Program

Specialty: General Surgery

Program name: Medical College of Georgia Program

Program code: 440-12-31-082

NRMP Code: 1985440C0, 1985440P0

Program type: University-based

State: Georgia

Address: Georgia Regents University Medical College of Georgia

1120 15th St, Augusta, GA 30912-4000

Phone: (706) 721-2503

Fax: (706) 721-1047

Percentage of IMGs in the program: 10%

Minimum USMLE Step 1 Score Requirement: 220
Minimum USMLE Step 2 Score Requirement: 220
Attempts on any step: Must pass on first attempt
CS required at time of application: No
USCE Requirement: None
Cut-Off time since graduation: No limits set
Program offers couple match: Yes
Visas Sponsored or accepted: J1 visa

Atlanta Medical Center General Surgery Residency Program

Specialty: General Surgery
Program name: Atlanta Medical Center Program
Program code: 440-12-22-080
NRMP Code: 1112440P0, 1112440C0
Program type: Community-based
State: Georgia
Address: Atlanta Medical Center
          303 Parkway Dr NE, Atlanta, GA 30312
Phone: (404) 265-4411
Fax: (404) 265-4989
Percentage of IMGs in the program: 0%
Minimum USMLE Step 1 Score Requirement: No limits set

Minimum USMLE Step 2 Score Requirement: No limits set

Attempts on any step: Must pass on first attempt except for CS exam where passing on 2nd attempt is allowed

CS required at time of application: Yes including ECFMG certificate

USCE Requirement: None

Cut-Off time since graduation: No limits set

Program offers couple match: Yes

Visas Sponsored or accepted: No visa

Morehouse School of Medicine General Surgery Residency Program

Specialty: General Surgery

Program name: Morehouse School of Medicine Program

Program code: 440-12-21-397

NRMP Code: 2099440P0, 2099440C0

Program type: Community-based university affiliated hospital

State: Georgia

Address: Morehouse School of Medicine
720 Westview Dr SW, Atlanta, GA 30310-1495

Phone: (404) 616-1426

Fax: (404) 616-6281
Percentage of IMGs in the program: 10%
Minimum USMLE Step 1 Score Requirement: 215
Minimum USMLE Step 2 Score Requirement: 215
Attempts on any step: Must pass on first attempt on any exam except CS exam where passing on the 2nd attempt allowed
CS required at time of application: Yes including ECFMG certificate
USCE Requirement: None
Cut-Off time since graduation: No limits set
Program offers couple match: Yes
Visas Sponsored or accepted: J1 visa

Medical Center of Central Georgia/Mercer University School of Medicine General Surgery Residency Program

Specialty: General Surgery
Program name: Medical Center of Central Georgia/Mercer University School of Medicine Program
Program code: 440-12-21-083
NRMP Code: 1120440C0
Program type: Community-based university affiliated hospital
State: Georgia

Address: Medical Center of Central Georgia
          777 Hemlock St, Macon, GA 31201
Phone: (478) 633-8101
Fax: (478) 633-5153
Percentage of IMGs in the program: 0%
Minimum USMLE Step 1 Score Requirement:
No limits set
Minimum USMLE Step 2 Score Requirement:
No limits set
Attempts on any step: Must pass on first
attempt on any step including CS exam
CS required at time of application: Yes
including ECFMG certificate
USCE Requirement: None
Cut-Off time since graduation: 1 year
Program offers couple match: Yes
Visas Sponsored or accepted: No visa

Emory University General Surgery Residency Program

Specialty: General Surgery
Program name: Emory University Program
Program code: 440-12-21-079
NRMP Code: 1113440C0, 1113440P0
Program type: University-based
State: Georgia
Address: Emory University Hospital
          1364 Clifton Rd NE, Atlanta, GA 30322
Phone: (404) 727-0093

Fax: (404) 712-0561
Percentage of IMGs in the program: 10%
Minimum USMLE Step 1 Score Requirement: 230
Minimum USMLE Step 2 Score Requirement: 230
Attempts on any step: Must pass on first attempt
CS required at time of application: No
USCE Requirement: None
Cut-Off time since graduation: 3 years
Program offers couple match: Yes
Visas Sponsored or accepted: J1 visa

Hawaii

University of Hawaii General Surgery Residency Program

Specialty: General Surgery
Program name: University of Hawaii Program
Program code: 440-14-21-085
NRMP Code: 3350440C0, 3350440P0
Program type: Community-based university

affiliated hospital
State: Hawaii
Address: University of Hawaii John A Burns
School of Medicine
          1356 Lusitana St, Honolulu, HI 96813-
2478
Phone: (808) 586-2920
Fax: (808) 586-3022
Percentage of IMGs in the program: 5%
Minimum USMLE Step 1 Score Requirement:
No limits set
Minimum USMLE Step 2 Score Requirement:
No limits set
Attempts on any step: Must pass on first
attempt
CS required at time of application: Yes
including ECFMG certificate
USCE Requirement: None
Cut-Off time since graduation: No limits set
Program offers couple match: Yes
Visas Sponsored or accepted: J1 visa

Illinois

Carle Foundation Hospital General Surgery Residency Program

Specialty: General Surgery
Program name: Carle Foundation Hospital Program
Program code: 440-16-12-430
NRMP Code: 1226440P0, 1226440C0
Program type: Community-based university affiliated hospital
State: Illinois
Address: Carle Foundation Hospital, Graduate Med Education GSRP
      611 W Park St, Urbana, IL 61801
Phone: (217) 383-6933
Fax: (217) 326-1300
Percentage of IMGs in the program: 0%
Minimum USMLE Step 1 Score Requirement: No limits set
Minimum USMLE Step 2 Score Requirement: No limits set
Attempts on any step: Must pass on first attempt including CS exam
CS required at time of application: Yes including ECFMG certificate
USCE Requirement: Yes
Cut-Off time since graduation: 3 years
Program offers couple match: No
Visas Sponsored or accepted: No visa

University of Chicago General Surgery Residency Program

Specialty: General Surgery
Program name: University of Chicago Program
Program code: 440-16-11-094
NRMP Code: 1160440P1, 1160440C0, 1160440P2
Program type: University-based
State: Illinois
Address: University of Chicago Hospitals, MC-6040,

5841 S Maryland Ave, Chicago, IL 60637-1470
Phone: (773) 702-6337
Fax: (773) 702-2140
Percentage of IMGs in the program: 6%
Minimum USMLE Step 1 Score Requirement: No limits set
Minimum USMLE Step 2 Score Requirement: No limits set
Attempts on any step: No limits set
CS required at time of application: No
USCE Requirement: None
Cut-Off time since graduation: 5 years
Program offers couple match: Yes
Visas Sponsored or accepted: J1 visa

McGaw Medical Center of Northwestern University General Surgery Residency Program

Specialty: General Surgery
Program name: McGaw Medical Center of Northwestern University Program
Program code: 440-16-21-091
State: Illinois
Address: McGaw Medical Center Northwestern University, Galter 3-150,
            251 E Huron St, Chicago, IL 60611-2950
Phone: (312) 926-9404
Fax: (312) 695-9194
Percentage of IMGs in the program: 0%
Minimum USMLE Step 1 Score Requirement: No limits set
Minimum USMLE Step 2 Score Requirement: No limits set
Attempts on any step: No limits set
CS required at time of application: No
USCE Requirement: None
Cut-Off time since graduation: No limits set
Program offers couple match: Yes
Visas Sponsored or accepted: J1 visa

Rush University Medical Center General Surgery Residency Program

Specialty: General Surgery
Program name: Rush University Medical Center Program
Program code: 440-16-21-092
Program type: University-based
State: Illinois
Address: Rush University Medical Center, Department of Surgery,
1653 W Congress Pkwy, Chicago, IL 60612
Phone: (312) 942-6510
Fax: (312) 942-2867
Percentage of IMGs in the program: 10%
Minimum USMLE Step 1 Score Requirement: No limits set
Minimum USMLE Step 2 Score Requirement: No limits set
Attempts on any step: No limits set
CS required at time of application: Yes including ECFMG certificate
USCE Requirement: None
Cut-Off time since graduation: 5 years
Program offers couple match: Yes
Visas Sponsored or accepted: J1 visa and H1b visa

Loyola University General Surgery Residency Program

Specialty: General Surgery
Program name: Loyola University Program
Program code: 440-16-21-099
NRMP Code: 1170440C0, 1170440P2, 1170440P0
Program type: University-based
State: Illinois
Address: Loyola University Medical Center, Department of Surgery EMS-3210,
          2160 S First Ave, Maywood, IL 60153
Phone: (708) 327-3436
Fax: (708) 327-3489
Percentage of IMGs in the program: 8%
Minimum USMLE Step 1 Score Requirement: 220
Minimum USMLE Step 2 Score Requirement: 220
Attempts on any step: No limits set
CS required at time of application: No
USCE Requirement: Yes, 12 months
Cut-Off time since graduation: No limits set
Program offers couple match: Yes
Visas Sponsored or accepted: J1 visa

University of Illinois College of Medicine at Peoria General Surgery Residency Program

Specialty: General Surgery
Program name: University of Illinois College of Medicine at Peoria Program
Program code: 440-16-21-101
NRMP Code: 1175440C0
Program type: Community-based university affiliated hospital
State: Illinois
Address: University of Illinois College of Medicine-Peoria,

   Department of Surgery 2nd Floor,
   624 NE Glen Oak Ave, Peoria, IL 61603
Phone: (309) 655-4775
Fax: (309) 655-3630
Percentage of IMGs in the program: 10%
Minimum USMLE Step 1 Score Requirement: No limits set
Minimum USMLE Step 2 Score Requirement: No limits set
Attempts on any step: No limits set
CS required at time of application: No
USCE Requirement: At least 1 year in surgery for IMGs (like prelim)
Cut-Off time since graduation: No limits set
Program offers couple match: Yes
Visas Sponsored or accepted: J1 visa and H1b visa

Southern Illinois University General Surgery Residency Program

Specialty: General Surgery
Program name: Southern Illinois University Program
Program code: 440-16-21-102
NRMP Code: 2922440P2, 2922440C0
Program type: University-based
State: Illinois
Address: Southern Illinois University School of Medicine, PO Box 19638,
       701 N First St, Springfield, IL 62794-9638
Phone: (217) 545-4401
Fax: (217) 545-2529
Percentage of IMGs in the program: 8%
Minimum USMLE Step 1 Score Requirement: 210
Minimum USMLE Step 2 Score Requirement: No limits set
Attempts on any step: No limits set
CS required at time of application: No
USCE Requirement: None
Cut-Off time since graduation: No limits set
Program offers couple match: Yes
Visas Sponsored or accepted: J1 visa

University of Illinois College of Medicine at Chicago (Mount Sinai) General Surgery Residency Program

Specialty: General Surgery
Program name: University of Illinois College of Medicine at Chicago (Mount Sinai) Program
Program code: 440-16-21-385
NRMP Code: 1287440P0, 1287440C0
Program type: Community-based university affiliated hospital
State: Illinois
Address: Mount Sinai Hospital Medical Center, Department of Surgery F930,
            1500 S California Ave, Chicago, IL 60608
Phone: (773) 257-6464
Fax: (773) 257-6548
Percentage of IMGs in the program: 5%
Minimum USMLE Step 1 Score Requirement: 220
Minimum USMLE Step 2 Score Requirement: 220
Attempts on any step: No limits set
CS required at time of application: No
USCE Requirement: Yes, 6 months
Cut-Off time since graduation: 2 years
Program offers couple match: No

Visas Sponsored or accepted: J1 visa

University of Illinois College of Medicine at Chicago General Surgery Residency Program

Specialty: General Surgery
Program name: University of Illinois College of Medicine at Chicago Program
Program code: 440-16-21-395
NRMP Code: 1150440P0, 1150440P1, 1150440C0
Program type: University-based
State: Illinois
Address: University of Illinois Hospital
        Department of Surgery MC 958 Ste 376-CSN
        840 S Wood St, Chicago, IL 60612-7322
Phone: (312) 996-6765
Fax: (312) 355-3755
Percentage of IMGs in the program: 20%
Minimum USMLE Step 1 Score Requirement: 220
Minimum USMLE Step 2 Score Requirement: 220
Attempts on any step: Must pass on first attempt including CS exam

CS required at time of application: Yes
including ECFMG certificate
USCE Requirement: None
Cut-Off time since graduation: 5 years
Program offers couple match: Yes
Visas Sponsored or accepted: J1 visa

Presence St Joseph Hospital (Chicago) General Surgery Residency Program

Specialty: General Surgery
Program name: Presence St Joseph Hospital (Chicago) Program
Program code: 440-16-31-086
State: Illinois
Address: St Joseph Hospital, Department of Surgery,
          2900 N Lake Shore Dr, Chicago, IL 60657
Phone: (773) 665-6237
Percentage of IMGs in the program: 20%
Minimum USMLE Step 1 Score Requirement: 215
Minimum USMLE Step 2 Score Requirement: 215
Attempts on any step: Must pass on first attempt

CS required at time of application: No
USCE Requirement: None
Cut-Off time since graduation: 2 years
Program offers couple match: Yes
Visas Sponsored or accepted: J1 visa and H1b visa

University of Illinois College of Medicine at Chicago (Metropolitan Group) General Surgery Residency Program

Specialty: General Surgery
Program name: University of Illinois College of Medicine at Chicago (Metropolitan Group) Program
Program code: 440-16-31-096
NRMP Code: 2920440C0, 2920440P0
Program type: Community-based university affiliated hospital
State: Illinois
Address: Advocate Illinois Masonic Medical Center, Room 4807,
            836 W Wellington Ave, Chicago, IL 60657
Phone: (773) 296-5347
Fax: (773) 296-5570
Percentage of IMGs in the program: 25%
Minimum USMLE Step 1 Score Requirement: 222

Minimum USMLE Step 2 Score Requirement: 210
Attempts on any step: Must pass on first attempt including CS exam
CS required at time of application: Yes including ECFMG certificate
USCE Requirement: None
Cut-Off time since graduation: No limits set
Program offers couple match: Yes
Visas Sponsored or accepted: J1 visa

Indiana

Indiana University School of Medicine General Surgery Residency Program

Specialty: General Surgery
Program name: Indiana University School of Medicine Program
Program code: 440-17-21-103
NRMP Code: 1187440C0, 1187440P0
Program type: Community-based university affiliated hospital
State: Indiana
Address: Indiana University School of Medicine, Emerson Hall 202,
545 Barnhill Dr, Indianapolis, IN 46202

Phone: (317) 274-4966
Fax: (317) 274-8769
Percentage of IMGs in the program: 10%
Minimum USMLE Step 1 Score Requirement: 220
Minimum USMLE Step 2 Score Requirement: 220
Attempts on any step: Must pass on first attempt
CS required at time of application: No
USCE Requirement: None
Cut-Off time since graduation: 3 years
Program offers couple match: Yes
Visas Sponsored or accepted: J1 visa

St Vincent Hospitals and Health Care Center General Surgery Residency Program

Specialty: General Surgery
Program name: St Vincent Hospitals and Health Care Center Program
Program code: 440-17-00-437
State: Indiana
Address: St Vincent Hospital and Health Care Center, General Surgery Program,
        2001 W 86th St, Indianapolis, IN 46260
Phone: (317) 338-6811

Fax:
Percentage of IMGs in the program: 40%
Minimum USMLE Step 1 Score Requirement: 220
Minimum USMLE Step 2 Score Requirement: 220
Attempts on any step: Must pass on first attempt
CS required at time of application: No
USCE Requirement: None
Cut-Off time since graduation: 3 years
Program offers couple match: Yes
Visas Sponsored or accepted: J1 visa

Iowa

Mercy Hospital Medical Center General Surgery Residency Program

Specialty: General Surgery
Program name: Mercy Hospital Medical Center Program
Program code: 440-18-00-436
Program type: Community-based university affiliated hospital

State: Iowa
Address: Mercy Hospital Medical Center, Surgery Program,
         1111 6th Ave, Des Moines, IA 50314-2611
Phone: (515) 643-2261
Fax: (515) 643-5802
Percentage of IMGs in the program: 0%
Minimum USMLE Step 1 Score Requirement: 210
Minimum USMLE Step 2 Score Requirement: 210
Attempts on any step: Must pass on maximum 2nd attempt
CS required at time of application: Yes including ECFMG certificate
USCE Requirement: 3 months
Cut-Off time since graduation: 3 years unless clinically active
Program offers couple match: Yes
Visas Sponsored or accepted: J1 visa

University of Iowa Hospitals and Clinics General Surgery Residency Program

Specialty: General Surgery
Program name: University of Iowa Hospitals and Clinics Program

Program code: 440-18-21-107
State: Iowa
Address: University of Iowa Hospitals and Clinics, Department of Surgery 1527 JCP,
200 Hawkins Dr, Iowa City, IA 52242-1086
Phone: (319) 353-6425
Fax: (319) 356-8682
Percentage of IMGs in the program: 5%
Minimum USMLE Step 1 Score Requirement: No limits set
Minimum USMLE Step 2 Score Requirement: No limits set
Attempts on any step: No limits set
CS required at time of application: No
USCE Requirement: None
Cut-Off time since graduation: No limits set
Program offers couple match: Yes
Visas Sponsored or accepted: J1 visa and H1b visa

Central Iowa Health System (Iowa Methodist Medical Center) General Surgery Residency Program

Specialty: General Surgery
Program name: Central Iowa Health System (Iowa Methodist Medical Center) Program
Program code: 440-18-22-105
NRMP Code: 1201440C0, 1201440P0

Program type: Community-based university affiliated hospital
State: Iowa
Address: Iowa Methodist Medical Center, Department of Surgery Suite 140,
   1415 Woodland Ave, Des Moines, IA 50309-1453
Phone: (515) 241-4078
Fax: (515) 241-4080
Percentage of IMGs in the program: 0%
Minimum USMLE Step 1 Score Requirement: No limits set
Minimum USMLE Step 2 Score Requirement: No limits set
Attempts on any step: Must pass on maximum 2nd attempt
CS required at time of application: Yes including ECFMG certificate
USCE Requirement: 1 year
Cut-Off time since graduation: 2 years
Program offers couple match: Yes
Visas Sponsored or accepted: J1 visa

Kansas

University of Kansas School of Medicine General Surgery Residency Program

Specialty: General Surgery
Program name: University of Kansas School of Medicine Program
Program code: 440-19-21-108
NRMP Code:
Program type:
State: Kansas
Address: University of Kansas Medical Center, Department of Surgery,
      3901 Rainbow Blvd, Kansas City, KS 66160
Phone: (913) 588-6124
Fax: (913) 588-7540
Percentage of IMGs in the program: 0%
Minimum USMLE Step 1 Score Requirement: 210
Minimum USMLE Step 2 Score Requirement: 210
Attempts on any step: Must pass on first atempt
CS required at time of application: No
USCE Requirement: None
Cut-Off time since graduation: 2 years
Program offers couple match: Yes
Visas Sponsored or accepted: J1 visa

University of Kansas (Wichita) General Surgery Residency Program

Specialty: General Surgery
Program name: University of Kansas (Wichita) Program
Program code: 440-19-21-387
NRMP Code: 3054440P0, 3054440C0
Program type: Community-based university affiliated hospital
State: Kansas
Address: Via Christi Regional Medical Center, Department of Surgery Room 3082, 929 N St Francis, Wichita, KS 67214
Phone: (316) 268-5990
Fax: (316) 291-7662
Percentage of IMGs in the program: 0%
Minimum USMLE Step 1 Score Requirement: 220
Minimum USMLE Step 2 Score Requirement: 220
Attempts on any step: Must pass on first attempt
CS required at time of application: No
USCE Requirement: Yes at least 1 month
Cut-Off time since graduation: 5 years
Program offers couple match: Yes
Visas Sponsored or accepted: J1 visa

Kentucky

University of Kentucky College of Medicine General Surgery Residency Program

Specialty: General Surgery
Program name: University of Kentucky College of Medicine Program
Program code:440-20-21-112
NRMP Code: 1848440P4, 1848440P1, 1848440C0, 1848440P0
Program type: University-based
State: Kentucky
Address: University of Kentucky Medical Center, Division of General Surgery C246, 800 Rose St, Lexington, KY 40536-0293
Phone: (859) 323-6762
Fax: (859) 323-6840
Percentage of IMGs in the program: 0%
Minimum USMLE Step 1 Score Requirement: No limits set
Minimum USMLE Step 2 Score Requirement: No limits set
Attempts on any step: Must pass on first attempt
CS required at time of application: No
USCE Requirement: None

Cut-Off time since graduation: 4 years
Program offers couple match: Yes
Visas Sponsored or accepted: J1 visa

University of Louisville General Surgery Residency Program

Specialty: General Surgery
Program name: University of Louisville Program
Program code: 440-20-21-113
Program type: University-based
State: Kentucky
Address: University of Louisville Hospital, Department of Surgery,
          550 S Jackson St, Louisville, KY 40292
Phone: (502) 852-6191
Fax: (502) 852-8915
Percentage of IMGs in the program: 0%
Minimum USMLE Step 1 Score Requirement: No limits set
Minimum USMLE Step 2 Score Requirement: No limits set
Attempts on any step: Must pass on first attempt
CS required at time of application: Yes including ECFMG certificate
USCE Requirement: None
Cut-Off time since graduation: No limits set
Program offers couple match: Yes
Visas Sponsored or accepted: J1 visa

Louisiana

Louisiana State University General Surgery Residency Program

Specialty: General Surgery
Program name: Louisiana State University Program
Program code: 440-21-21-114
NRMP Code: 1224440P3, 1224440C0, 1224440P2
Program type: University-based
State: Louisiana
Address: LSU Health Science Center New Orleans, Department of Surgery Room 734, 1542 Tulane Ave, New Orleans, LA 70112-2822
Phone: (504) 568-4760
Fax: (504) 568-4633
Percentage of IMGs in the program: 10%
Minimum USMLE Step 1 Score Requirement: 210
Minimum USMLE Step 2 Score Requirement: 210
Attempts on any step: Must pass on first attempt
CS required at time of application: Yes

USCE Requirement: None
Cut-Off time since graduation: No limits set
Program offers couple match: Yes
Visas Sponsored or accepted: H1b visa

Louisiana State University (Shreveport) General Surgery Residency Program

Specialty: General Surgery
Program name: Louisiana State University (Shreveport) Program
Program code: 440-21-21-117
NRMP Code: 1232440C0, 1232440P0
Program type: University-based
State: Louisiana
Address: LSU Health Science Center Shreveport, PO Box 33932,
          1501 Kings Hwy, Shreveport, LA 71103
Phone: (318) 675-6111
Fax: (318) 675-6141
Percentage of IMGs in the program: 0%
Minimum USMLE Step 1 Score Requirement: 230
Minimum USMLE Step 2 Score Requirement: 230
Attempts on any step: Must pass on first attempt
CS required at time of application: No

USCE Requirement: None
Cut-Off time since graduation: 3 years
Program offers couple match: Yes
Visas Sponsored or accepted: J1 visa

Tulane University General Surgery Residency Program

Specialty: General Surgery
Program name: Tulane University Program
Program code: 440-21-21-423
NRMP Code: 3073440C0, 3073440P0, 3073440P1
Program type: University-based
State: Louisiana
Address: Tulane University Health Sciences Center, Department of Surgery SL22,
          1430 Tulane Ave, New Orleans, LA 70112
Phone: (504) 988-2306
Fax: (504) 988-1882
Percentage of IMGs in the program: 0%
Minimum USMLE Step 1 Score Requirement: No limits set
Minimum USMLE Step 2 Score Requirement: No limits set
Attempts on any step: No limits set
CS required at time of application: No
USCE Requirement: Yes, at least 1 month

Cut-Off time since graduation: No limits set
Program offers couple match: Yes
Visas Sponsored or accepted: J1 visa

Ochsner Clinic Foundation General Surgery Residency Program

Specialty: General Surgery
Program name: Ochsner Clinic Foundation Program
Program code: 440-21-22-115
NRMP Code: 1966440C0, 1966440P0
Program type: Community-based
State: Louisiana
Address: Ochsner Clinic Foundation, GME Office,
        1514 Jefferson Hwy, New Orleans, LA 70121
Phone: (504) 842-6829
Fax: (504) 842-0089
Percentage of IMGs in the program: 5%
Minimum USMLE Step 1 Score Requirement: 220
Minimum USMLE Step 2 Score Requirement: 220
Attempts on any step: Must pass on first attempt including CS exam
CS required at time of application: No
USCE Requirement: Yes
Cut-Off time since graduation: 5 years

Program offers couple match: Yes
Visas Sponsored or accepted: J1 visa

Maine

Maine Medical Center General Surgery Residency Program

Specialty: General Surgery
Program name: Maine Medical Center Program
Program code: 440-22-21-119
NRMP Code: 1236440P0, 1236440P1, 1236440C0
Program type: Community-based university affiliated hospital
State: Maine
Address: Maine Medical Center, Department of Surgery,
          22 Bramhall St, Portland, ME 04102-3175
Phone: (207) 662-4078
Fax: (207) 662-6389
Percentage of IMGs in the program: 10%
Minimum USMLE Step 1 Score Requirement: 220
Minimum USMLE Step 2 Score Requirement: 220

Attempts on any step: Must pass on first attempt
CS required at time of application: Yes
USCE Requirement: None
Cut-Off time since graduation: No limits set
Program offers couple match: Yes
Visas Sponsored or accepted: J1 visa

Maryland

Union Memorial Hospital General Surgery Residency Program

Specialty: General Surgery
Program name: Union Memorial Hospital Program
Program code: 440-23-21-127
NRMP Code: 1251440P0, 1251440C0
Program type: Community-based university affiliated hospital
State: Maryland
Address: Union Memorial Hospital, Surgery Program,
201 E University Pkwy, Baltimore, MD 21218
Phone: (410) 554-2782
Fax: (410) 261-8085
Percentage of IMGs in the program: 20%

Minimum USMLE Step 1 Score Requirement: 220

Minimum USMLE Step 2 Score Requirement: 220

Attempts on any step: Must pass on first attempt

CS required at time of application: Yes including ECFMG certificate

USCE Requirement: None

Cut-Off time since graduation: 2 years

Program offers couple match: No

Visas Sponsored or accepted: J1 visa

University of Maryland General Surgery Residency Program

Specialty: General Surgery

Program name: University of Maryland Program

Program code: 440-23-21-128

NRMP Code: 1252440C0, 1252440P0, 1252440P2

Program type: University-based

State: Maryland

Address: University of Maryland Medical System, Department of Surgery,
22 S Greene St, Baltimore, MD 21201

Phone: (410) 328-5878

Fax: (410) 328-5919

Percentage of IMGs in the program: 10%

Minimum USMLE Step 1 Score Requirement:
No limits set
Minimum USMLE Step 2 Score Requirement:
No limits set
Attempts on any step: No limits set
CS required at time of application: Yes
including ECFMG certificate
USCE Requirement: None
Cut-Off time since graduation: 10 years but
prefer less than 5 years
Program offers couple match: Yes
Visas Sponsored or accepted: J1 visa

Johns Hopkins University General Surgery Residency Program

Specialty: General Surgery
Program name: Johns Hopkins University
Program
Program code: 440-23-21-392
NRMP Code: 1242440C0, 1242440P0
Program type: University-based
State: Maryland
Address: Johns Hopkins School of Medicine,
        Department of Surgery Blalock 658,
        600 N Wolfe St, Baltimore, MD 21287
Phone: (410) 955-6796
Fax: (410) 955-0834
Percentage of IMGs in the program: 10%

Minimum USMLE Step 1 Score Requirement: 220

Minimum USMLE Step 2 Score Requirement: 220

Attempts on any step: No limits set

CS required at time of application: Yes including ECFMG certificate

USCE Requirement: None

Cut-Off time since graduation: No limits set

Program offers couple match: Yes

Visas Sponsored or accepted: J1 visa

Sinai Hospital of Baltimore General Surgery Residency Program

Specialty: General Surgery

Program name: Sinai Hospital of Baltimore Program

Program code: 440-23-21-417

NRMP Code: 1249440C0

Program type: Community-based university affiliated hospital

State: Maryland

Address: Sinai Hospital of Baltimore, Hoffberger Professional Building Suite 42,
        2435 W Belvedere Ave, Baltimore, MD 21215

Phone: (410) 601-6412

Fax: (410) 601-5835
Percentage of IMGs in the program: 60%
Minimum USMLE Step 1 Score Requirement: 215
Minimum USMLE Step 2 Score Requirement: 215
Attempts on any step: Must pass maximum on the 2nd attempt
CS required at time of application: No
USCE Requirement: Yes
Cut-Off time since graduation: No limits set
Program offers couple match: Yes
Visas Sponsored or accepted: J1 visa

St Agnes HealthCare General Surgery Residency Program

Specialty: General Surgery
Program name: St Agnes HealthCare Program
Program code: 440-23-22-123
NRMP Code: 1247440P0, 1247440C0
Program type: Community-based university affiliated hospital
State: Maryland
Address: St Agnes HealthCare, Department of Surgery Box 207,
          900 Caton Ave, Baltimore, MD 21229-5299
Phone: (410) 368-2718

Fax: (410) 951-4007
Percentage of IMGs in the program: 50%
Minimum USMLE Step 1 Score Requirement: 225
Minimum USMLE Step 2 Score Requirement: 225
Attempts on any step: Must pass from first attempt
CS required at time of application: Yes including ECFMG certificate
USCE Requirement: None
Cut-Off time since graduation: 5 years
Program offers couple match: Yes
Visas Sponsored or accepted: J1 visa

Massachusetts

Baystate Medical Center/Tufts University School of Medicine General Surgery Residency Program

Specialty: General Surgery
Program name: Baystate Medical Center/Tufts University School of Medicine Program

Program code: 440-24-11-138
NRMP Code: 1286440C0, 1286440P0
Program type: Community-based university affiliated hospital
State: Massachusetts
Address: Baystate Medical Center, Department of Surgical Education S3653,
            759 Chestnut St, Springfield, MA 01199
Phone: (413) 794-5165
Fax: (413) 794-1835
Percentage of IMGs in the program: 20%
Minimum USMLE Step 1 Score Requirement: No limits set
Minimum USMLE Step 2 Score Requirement: No limits set
Attempts on any step: Must pass on first attempt
CS required at time of application: Yes including ECFMG certificate
USCE Requirement: Yes, 6 months
Cut-Off time since graduation: 2 years
Program offers couple match: Yes
Visas Sponsored or accepted: J1 visa

Boston Medical Center General Surgery Residency Program

Specialty: General Surgery

Program name: Boston Medical Center Program
Program code: 440-24-21-131
State: Massachusetts
Address: Boston University Medical Center, Surgery Program Room C515,
          88 E Newton St, Boston, MA 02118-2393
Phone: (617) 638-8442
Fax: (617) 638-8409
Percentage of IMGs in the program: 5%
Minimum USMLE Step 1 Score Requirement: No limits set
Minimum USMLE Step 2 Score Requirement: No limits set
Attempts on any step: No limits set
CS required at time of application: Yes including ECFMG certificate
USCE Requirement: None
Cut-Off time since graduation: No limits set
Program offers couple match: Yes
Visas Sponsored or accepted: J1 visa and H1b visa

Tufts Medical Center General Surgery Residency Program

Specialty: General Surgery
Program name: Tufts Medical Center Program
Program code: 440-24-21-134
NRMP Code: 1263440C0, 1263440P0

Program type: University-based
State: Massachusetts
Address: Tufts Medical Center, Box 437,
        800 Washington St, Boston, MA
02111
Phone: (617) 636-5891
Fax: (617) 636-5498
Percentage of IMGs in the program: 30%
Minimum USMLE Step 1 Score Requirement:
230
Minimum USMLE Step 2 Score Requirement:
230
Attempts on any step: No limits set
CS required at time of application: Yes
including ECFMG certificate
USCE Requirement: Yes, 3 months
Cut-Off time since graduation: 2 years
Program offers couple match: Yes
Visas Sponsored or accepted: J1 visa

Brigham and Women's Hospital General Surgery Residency Program

Specialty: General Surgery
Program name: Brigham and Women's Hospital
Program
Program code: 440-24-21-135
NRMP Code: 1265440C0, 1265440P0

State: Massachusetts
Address: Brigham and Women's Hospital, CA-034,

       75 Francis St, Boston, MA 02115
Phone: (617) 732-6861
Fax: (617) 264-6850
Percentage of IMGs in the program: 5%
Minimum USMLE Step 1 Score Requirement: No limits set
Minimum USMLE Step 2 Score Requirement: No limits set
Attempts on any step: No limits set
CS required at time of application: Yes including ECFMG certificate
USCE Requirement: None
Cut-Off time since graduation: No limits set
Program offers couple match: Yes
Visas Sponsored or accepted: No visa

St Elizabeth's Medical Center General Surgery Residency Program

Specialty: General Surgery
Program name: St Elizabeth's Medical Center Program
Program code: 440-24-21-136
NRMP Code: 1266440C0
Program type: Community-based university affiliated hospital

State: Massachusetts
Address: St Elizabeth's Medical Center, CMP2,
                    736 Cambridge St, Boston, MA 02135
Phone: (617) 789-2990
Fax: (617) 789-3419
Percentage of IMGs in the program: 10%
Minimum USMLE Step 1 Score Requirement:
220
Minimum USMLE Step 2 Score Requirement:
220
Attempts on any step: Must pass on first
attempt
CS required at time of application: Yes
including ECFMG certificate
USCE Requirement: None
Cut-Off time since graduation: No limits set
Program offers couple match: Yes
Visas Sponsored or accepted: J1 visa

University of Massachusetts General Surgery Residency Program

Specialty: General Surgery
Program name: University of Massachusetts
Program
Program code: 440-24-21-139
NRMP Code: 3050440P0, 3050440C0
Program type: University-based
State: Massachusetts

Address: University of Massachusetts Medical School, Department of Surgery,

55 Lake Ave N, Worcester, MA 01655

Phone: (508) 856-3744

Fax: (508) 334-3306

Percentage of IMGs in the program: 10%

Minimum USMLE Step 1 Score Requirement: 220

Minimum USMLE Step 2 Score Requirement: 220

Attempts on any step: Must pass on first attempt

CS required at time of application: Yes including ECFMG certificate

USCE Requirement: Yes, 6 months

Cut-Off time since graduation: 3 years

Program offers couple match: Yes

Visas Sponsored or accepted: J1 visa

Lahey Clinic General Surgery Residency Program

Specialty: General Surgery

Program name: Lahey Clinic Program

Program code: 440-24-21-401

NRMP Code: 3130440C0, 3130440P0

Program type: Community-based university affiliated hospital

State: Massachusetts

Address: Lahey Clinic, Department of General

Surgery,
41 Mall Road, Burlington, MA 01805
Phone: (781) 744-8193
Fax: (781) 744-3646
Percentage of IMGs in the program: 10%
Minimum USMLE Step 1 Score Requirement: 215
Minimum USMLE Step 2 Score Requirement: 215
Attempts on any step: Must pass on first attempt
CS required at time of application: Yes including ECFMG certificate
USCE Requirement: 3 months with 3 US LOR
Cut-Off time since graduation: 2 years
Program offers couple match: Yes
Visas Sponsored or accepted: J1 visa

Massachusetts General Hospital General Surgery Residency Program

Specialty: General Surgery
Program name: Massachusetts General Hospital Program
Program code: 440-24-31-132
State: Massachusetts
Address: Massachusetts General Hospital, Surgical Program GRB 425,

55 Fruit St, Boston, MA 02114
Phone: (617) 726-2800
Fax: (617) 724-3499
Percentage of IMGs in the program: 20%
Minimum USMLE Step 1 Score Requirement:
No limits set
Minimum USMLE Step 2 Score Requirement:
No limits set
Attempts on any step: No limits set
CS required at time of application: Yes
including ECFMG certificate
USCE Requirement: None
Cut-Off time since graduation: 5 years
Program offers couple match: Yes
Visas Sponsored or accepted: J1 visa and H1b
visa

Berkshire Medical Center General Surgery Residency Program

Specialty: General Surgery
Program name: Berkshire Medical Center
Program
Program code: 440-24-31-137
NRMP Code: 1281440P0, 1281440C0
Program type: Community-based university
affiliated hospital
State: Massachusetts
Address: Berkshire Medical Center, Surgery

Program,
                725 North St, Pittsfield, MA 01201
Phone: (413) 447-2741   Ext: 2
Fax: (413) 447-2766
Percentage of IMGs in the program: 70%
Minimum USMLE Step 1 Score Requirement: 220
Minimum USMLE Step 2 Score Requirement: 220
Attempts on any step: Must pass on first attempt, 2nd attempt might be looked at.
CS required at time of application: Yes including ECFMG certificate
USCE Requirement: None
Cut-Off time since graduation: 5 years
Program offers couple match: Yes
Visas Sponsored or accepted: J1 visa

Beth Israel Deaconess Medical Center General Surgery Residency Program

Specialty: General Surgery
Program name: Beth Israel Deaconess Medical Center Program
Program code: 440-24-31-409
NRMP Code: 1256440C0, 1256440P0
Program type: University-based
State: Massachusetts
Address: Beth Israel Deaconess Medical Center,

LMOB 9B,

330 Brookline Ave, Boston, MA 02215

Phone: (617) 632-9236

Fax: (617) 632-7424

Percentage of IMGs in the program: 20%

Minimum USMLE Step 1 Score Requirement:
No limits set

Minimum USMLE Step 2 Score Requirement:
No limits set

Attempts on any step: No limits set

CS required at time of application: Yes
including ECFMG certificate

USCE Requirement: None

Cut-Off time since graduation: No limits set

Program offers couple match: Yes

Visas Sponsored or accepted: J1 visa

Michigan

St Joseph Mercy Hospital General Surgery Residency Program

Specialty: General Surgery

Program name: St Joseph Mercy Hospital
Program

Program code: 440-25-11-140

NRMP code: 1292440C0
State: Michigan
Address: St Joseph Mercy Hospital
5333 McAuley Dr, Ann Arbor, MI 48106
Phone: (734) 712-7352
Fax: (734) 712-2054
Percentage of IMGs in the program: 10%
Minimum USMLE Step 1 Score Requirement: 210
Minimum USMLE Step 2 Score Requirement: 210
Attempts on any step: Must pass on first attempt
CS required at time of application: No
USCE Requirement: Yes, 2 months
Cut-Off time since graduation: Prefer less than 2 years
Program offers couple match: Yes
Visas Sponsored or accepted: J1 visa

St John Hospital and Medical Center General Surgery Residency Program

Specialty: General Surgery
Program name: St John Hospital and Medical Center Program
Program code: 440-25-11-145
NRMP Code: 1915440C0, 1915440P0

Program type: Community-based university affiliated hospital
State: Michigan
Address: St John Hospital and Medical Center
22101 Moross Rd, Detroit, MI 48236
Phone: (313) 343-3875
Fax: (313) 343-7840
Percentage of IMGs in the program: 15%
Minimum USMLE Step 1 Score Requirement: 210
Minimum USMLE Step 2 Score Requirement: 210
Attempts on any step: Must pass from first attempt
CS required at time of application: No
USCE Requirement: None
Cut-Off time since graduation: 5 years
Program offers couple match: Yes
Visas Sponsored or accepted: J1 visa and H1b visa

St Joseph Mercy-Oakland General Surgery Residency Program

Specialty: General Surgery
Program name: St Joseph Mercy-Oakland Program
Program code: 440-25-11-157
NRMP Code: 1319440C0, 1319440P0

Program type: Community-based university affiliated hospital
State: Michigan
Address: St Joseph Mercy-Oakland
        44405 Woodward Ave, Pontiac, MI 48341
Phone: (248) 858-3234
Fax: (248) 858-3244
Percentage of IMGs in the program: 30%
Minimum USMLE Step 1 Score Requirement: 220
Minimum USMLE Step 2 Score Requirement: 220
Attempts on any step: Must pass on first attempt
CS required at time of application: No
USCE Requirement: None
Cut-Off time since graduation: 2 years
Program offers couple match: Yes
Visas Sponsored or accepted: J1 visa

Henry Ford Hospital/Wayne State University General Surgery Residency Program

Specialty: General Surgery
Program name: Henry Ford Hospital/Wayne State University Program
Program code: 440-25-12-143
State: Michigan

Address: Henry Ford Hospital/Wayne State University
         2799 W Grand Blvd, Detroit, MI 48202
Phone: (313) 916-3056
Fax: (313) 916-5811
Percentage of IMGs in the program: 30%
Minimum USMLE Step 1 Score Requirement: 210
Minimum USMLE Step 2 Score Requirement: 210
Attempts on any step: Must pass on first attempt
CS required at time of application: No
USCE Requirement: None
Cut-Off time since graduation: No limits set
Program offers couple match: Yes
Visas Sponsored or accepted: J1 visa

William Beaumont Hospital General Surgery Residency Program

Specialty: General Surgery
Program name: William Beaumont Hospital Program
Program code: 440-25-12-158
State: Michigan
Address: William Beaumont Hospital
         3601 W 13 Mile Rd, Royal Oak, MI

48073
Phone: (248) 898-2674
Fax: (248) 898-1517
Percentage of IMGs in the program: 0%
Minimum USMLE Step 1 Score Requirement:
No limits set
Minimum USMLE Step 2 Score Requirement:
No limits set
Attempts on any step: No limits set
CS required at time of application: Yes
including ECFMG certificate
USCE Requirement: None
Cut-Off time since graduation: No limits set
Program offers couple match: Yes
Visas Sponsored or accepted: J1 visa and H1b
visa

University of Michigan General Surgery Residency Program

Specialty: General Surgery
Program name: University of Michigan Program
Program code: 440-25-21-141
NRMP Code: 1293440P0, 1293440C0,
1293440P2
Program type: University-based
State: Michigan
Address: University of Michigan Hospitals and
Health Centers
          1500 E Medical Center Dr, Ann Arbor,

MI 48109-5346
Phone: (734) 936-5732
Fax: (734) 936-5725
Percentage of IMGs in the program: 0%
Minimum USMLE Step 1 Score Requirement:
240
Minimum USMLE Step 2 Score Requirement:
240
Attempts on any step: Must pass on the first
attempt
CS required at time of application: Yes
including ECFMG certificate
USCE Requirement: None
Cut-Off time since graduation: prefer new
graduates
Program offers couple match: Yes
Visas Sponsored or accepted: J1 visa

Detroit Medical Center/Wayne State University General Surgery Residency Program

Specialty: General Surgery
Program name: Detroit Medical Center/Wayne
State University Program
Program code: 440-25-21-148
NRMP Code: 1295440C0, 1295440P0
Program type: Community-based university
affiliated hospital
State: Michigan

Address: Detroit Medical Center/Wayne State University
          4201 St Antoine Blvd, Detroit, MI 48201
Phone: (313) 577-5009
Fax: (313) 577-5310
Percentage of IMGs in the program: 20%
Minimum USMLE Step 1 Score Requirement: 215
Minimum USMLE Step 2 Score Requirement: 215
Attempts on any step: No limits set
CS required at time of application: Yes including ECFMG certificate
USCE Requirement: None
Cut-Off time since graduation: 3 years
Program offers couple match: Yes
Visas Sponsored or accepted: J1 visa

Providence Hospital and Medical Centers General Surgery Residency Program

Specialty: General Surgery
Program name: Providence Hospital and Medical Centers Program
Program code: 440-25-21-160
NRMP Code: 1303440P0, 1303440C0
Program type: Community-based university affiliated hospital

State: Michigan
Address: Providence Hospital and Medical Center
16001 W Nine Mile Rd, Southfield, MI 48075
Phone: (248) 849-3073
Fax: (248) 849-5380
Percentage of IMGs in the program: 60%
Minimum USMLE Step 1 Score Requirement: 210
Minimum USMLE Step 2 Score Requirement: 210
Attempts on any step: Must pass on first attempt
CS required at time of application: Yes including ECFMG certificate
USCE Requirement: Yes
Cut-Off time since graduation: 5 years
Program offers couple match: Yes
Visas Sponsored or accepted: J1 visa

Michigan State University General Surgery Residency Program

Specialty: General Surgery
Program name: Michigan State University Program
Program code: 440-25-21-386
NRMP Code: 2436440C0, 2436440P0
Program type: Community-based university

affiliated hospital
State: Michigan
Address: Sparrow Hospital
          1200 E Michigan Ave, Lansing, MI
48912-1837
Phone: (517) 267-2487
Fax: (517) 267-2488
Percentage of IMGs in the program: 0%
Minimum USMLE Step 1 Score Requirement:
220
Minimum USMLE Step 2 Score Requirement:
220
Attempts on any step: No limits set
CS required at time of application: No
USCE Requirement: None
Cut-Off time since graduation: Prefer recent
graduates
Program offers couple match: Yes
Visas Sponsored or accepted: J1 visa

Western Michigan University Homer Stryker MD School of Medicine General Surgery Residency Program

Specialty: General Surgery
Program name: Western Michigan University
Homer Stryker MD School of Medicine Program
Program code: 440-25-21-400
NRMP Code: 1314440C0, 1314440P0

Program type: University-based
State: Michigan
Address: Western Michigan University School of Medicine
             1000 Oakland Dr, Kalamazoo, MI 49008-1284
Phone: (269) 337-6256
Fax: (269) 337-6441
Percentage of IMGs in the program: 40%
Minimum USMLE Step 1 Score Requirement: 210
Minimum USMLE Step 2 Score Requirement: 210
Attempts on any step: Must pass on first attempt
CS required at time of application: Yes including ECFMG certificate
USCE Requirement: Yes
Cut-Off time since graduation: 3 years
Program offers couple match: Yes
Visas Sponsored or accepted: J1 visa and H1b visa

Grand Rapids Medical Education Partners/Michigan State University General Surgery Residency Program

Specialty: General Surgery

Program name: Grand Rapids Medical Education Partners/Michigan State University Program
Program code: 440-25-21-410
NRMP Code: 2077440C0, 2077440P0
Program type: Community-based university affiliated hospital
State: Michigan
Address: Grand Rapids Medical Education Partners
　　　221 Michigan St NE, Grand Rapids, MI 49503
Phone: (616) 391-1405
Fax: (616) 391-8611
Percentage of IMGs in the program: 0%
Minimum USMLE Step 1 Score Requirement: No limits set
Minimum USMLE Step 2 Score Requirement: No limits set
Attempts on any step: No limits set
CS required at time of application: Yes including ECFMG certificate
USCE Requirement: None
Cut-Off time since graduation: No limits set
Program offers couple match: Yes
Visas Sponsored or accepted: J1 visa

Minnesota

Hennepin County Medical Center General Surgery Residency Program

Specialty: General Surgery
Program name: Hennepin County Medical Center Program
Program code: 440-26-11-161
NRMP Code: 1329440P0, 1329440C0
Program type: Community-based
State: Minnesota
Address: Hennepin County Medical Center
          701 Park Ave S, Minneapolis, MN 55415
Phone: (612) 873-2849
Fax: (612) 904-4297
Percentage of IMGs in the program: 10% (variable)
Minimum USMLE Step 1 Score Requirement: 215
Minimum USMLE Step 2 Score Requirement: 215
Attempts on any step: Must pass on first attempt
CS required at time of application: Yes including ECFMG certificate
USCE Requirement: None
Cut-Off time since graduation: No limits set
Program offers couple match: Yes
Visas Sponsored or accepted: No visa

Mayo Clinic College of Medicine (Rochester) General Surgery Residency Program

Specialty: General Surgery
Program name: Mayo Clinic College of Medicine (Rochester) Program
Program code: 440-26-21-163
NRMP Code: 1328440P3, 1328440C0, 1328440P0
Program type: University-based
State: Minnesota
Address: Mayo Clinic
           200 First St SW, Rochester, MN 55905
Phone: (507) 284-4710
Fax: (507) 538-7288
Percentage of IMGs in the program: 50%
Minimum USMLE Step 1 Score Requirement: 220
Minimum USMLE Step 2 Score Requirement: 220
Attempts on any step: Must pass on first attempt
CS required at time of application: Yes including ECFMG certificate
USCE Requirement: None
Cut-Off time since graduation: 5 years
Program offers couple match: Yes
Visas Sponsored or accepted: J1 visa

University of Minnesota General Surgery Residency Program

Specialty: General Surgery
Program name: University of Minnesota Program
Program code: 440-26-31-162
NRMP Code: 1334440P0, 1334440C0
Program type: University-based
State: Minnesota
Address: University of Minnesota Medical Center
            420 Delaware St SE, Minneapolis, MN 55455-0321
Phone: (612) 626-2590
Fax: (612) 625-4411
Percentage of IMGs in the program: 10%
Minimum USMLE Step 1 Score Requirement: 220
Minimum USMLE Step 2 Score Requirement: 220
Attempts on any step: No limits set
CS required at time of application: Yes including ECFMG certificate
USCE Requirement: None
Cut-Off time since graduation: No limits set
Program offers couple match: Yes
Visas Sponsored or accepted: J1 visa

Mississippi

University of Mississippi Medical Center General Surgery Residency Program

Specialty: General Surgery
Program name: University of Mississippi Medical Center Program
Program code: 440-27-21-165
State: Mississippi
Address: University of Mississippi Medical Center
2500 N State St, Jackson, MS 39216-4505
Phone: (601) 984-5102
Fax: (601) 984-5110
Percentage of IMGs in the program: 15%
Minimum USMLE Step 1 Score Requirement: 200
Minimum USMLE Step 2 Score Requirement: 210
Attempts on any step: Must pass on the first attempt
CS required at time of application: Yes including ECFMG certificate
USCE Requirement: Yes
Cut-Off time since graduation: 5 years
Program offers couple match: Yes

Visas Sponsored or accepted: J1 visa

Missouri

University of Missouri-Columbia General Surgery Residency Program

Specialty: General Surgery
Program name: University of Missouri-Columbia Program
Program code: 440-28-21-166
NRMP Code: 1994440C0, 1994440P0, 1994440P1
Program type: University-based
State: Missouri
Address: University of Missouri Hospitals and Clinics

One Hospital Dr, Columbia, MO 65212
Phone: (573) 882-2245
Fax: (573) 884-4611
Percentage of IMGs in the program: 0%
Minimum USMLE Step 1 Score Requirement: No limits set
Minimum USMLE Step 2 Score Requirement: No limits set

Attempts on any step: No limits set
CS required at time of application: Yes
including ECFMG certificate
USCE Requirement: Yes
Cut-Off time since graduation: No limits set
Program offers couple match: Yes
Visas Sponsored or accepted: J1 visa and H1b
visa

University of Missouri at Kansas City General Surgery Residency Program

Specialty: General Surgery
Program name: University of Missouri at Kansas City Program
Program code: 440-28-21-168
NRMP Code: 1343440C0, 1343440P0
Program type: University-based
State: Missouri
Address: Truman Medical Center
         2301 Holmes St, Kansas City, MO 64108
Phone: (816) 404-5372
Fax: (816) 404-5381
Percentage of IMGs in the program: 10%
Minimum USMLE Step 1 Score Requirement: No limits set
Minimum USMLE Step 2 Score Requirement: No limits set

Attempts on any step: No limits set
CS required at time of application: No
USCE Requirement: None
Cut-Off time since graduation: No limits set
Program offers couple match: Yes
Visas Sponsored or accepted: No visa

St Louis University School of Medicine General Surgery Residency Program

Specialty: General Surgery
Program name: St Louis University School of Medicine Program
Program code: 440-28-21-171
NRMP Code: 1365440P0, 1365440C0
Program type: University-based
State: Missouri
Address: St Louis University School of Medicine
          3635 Vista Ave, St Louis, MO 63110-0250
Phone: (314) 577-8317   Ext: 4
Fax: (314) 268-5466
Percentage of IMGs in the program: 20%
Minimum USMLE Step 1 Score Requirement: No limits set
Minimum USMLE Step 2 Score Requirement: No limits set

Attempts on any step: Must pass on the first attempt
CS required at time of application: No
USCE Requirement: Yes
Cut-Off time since graduation: No limits set
Program offers couple match: Yes
Visas Sponsored or accepted: J1 visa

Washington University/B-JH/SLCH Consortium General Surgery Residency Program

Specialty: General Surgery
Program name: Washington University/B-JH/SLCH Consortium Program
Program code: 440-28-21-388
NRMP Code:
Program type:
State: Missouri
Address: Washington University Medical Center
          660 S Euclid Ave, St Louis, MO 63110
Phone: (314) 362-8028
Fax: (314) 747-1288
Percentage of IMGs in the program: 5%
Minimum USMLE Step 1 Score Requirement: No limits set
Minimum USMLE Step 2 Score Requirement: No limits set
Attempts on any step: Must pass on the first attempt

CS required at time of application: Yes
including ECFMG certificate
USCE Requirement: None
Cut-Off time since graduation: 5 years
Program offers couple match: Yes
Visas Sponsored or accepted: J1 visa

Nebraska

University of Nebraska Medical Center College of Medicine General Surgery Residency Program

Specialty: General Surgery
Program name: University of Nebraska Medical Center College of Medicine Program
Program code: 440-30-21-176
State: Nebraska
Address: University of Nebraska Medical Center
983280 Nebraska Medical Center,
Omaha, NE 68198-3280
Phone: (402) 559-5510
Fax: (402) 559-3356
Percentage of IMGs in the program: 20%
Minimum USMLE Step 1 Score Requirement: 220

Minimum USMLE Step 2 Score Requirement: 220
Attempts on any step: Must pass on the first attempt
CS required at time of application: Yes including ECFMG certificate
USCE Requirement: None
Cut-Off time since graduation: 5 years but must have clinical activity in the last 5 years
Program offers couple match: Yes
Visas Sponsored or accepted: J1 visa and H1b visa

Creighton University General Surgery Residency Program

Specialty: General Surgery
Program name: Creighton University Program
Program code: 440-30-31-175
NRMP Code: 1372440P0, 1372440C0
Program type: Community-based university affiliated hospital
State: Nebraska
Address: ACH Creighton University Medical Center
      601 N 30th St, Omaha, NE 68131
Phone: (402) 280-4669
Fax: (402) 280-4495
Percentage of IMGs in the program: 40%

Minimum USMLE Step 1 Score Requirement: 200

Minimum USMLE Step 2 Score Requirement: 210

Attempts on any step: No limits set

CS required at time of application: No

USCE Requirement: None

Cut-Off time since graduation: No limits set

Program offers couple match: Yes

Visas Sponsored or accepted: J1 visa

Nevada

University of Nevada School of Medicine (Las Vegas) General Surgery Residency Program

Specialty: General Surgery

Program name: University of Nevada School of Medicine (Las Vegas) Program

Program code: 440-31-21-378

NRMP Code: 2028440C0, 2028440P0

Program type: Community-based university affiliated hospital

State: Nevada

Address: University of Nevada School of Medicine
            2040 W Charleston Blvd, Las Vegas, NV 89102-2214
Phone: (702) 671-2273
Fax: (702) 385-9399
Percentage of IMGs in the program: 10% (variable)
Minimum USMLE Step 1 Score Requirement: 220
Minimum USMLE Step 2 Score Requirement: 220
Attempts on any step: Must pass on first attempt
CS required at time of application: Yes including ECFMG certificate
USCE Requirement: None
Cut-Off time since graduation: No limits set
Program offers couple match: Yes
Visas Sponsored or accepted: J1 visa

New Hampshire

Dartmouth-Hitchcock Medical Center General Surgery Residency Program

Specialty: General Surgery
Program name: Dartmouth-Hitchcock Medical Center Program
Program code: 440-32-21-177
NRMP Code: 1377440P0, 1377440P1, 1377440C0
Program type: University-based
State: New Hampshire
Address: Dartmouth-Hitchcock Medical Center One Medical Center Dr, Lebanon, NH 03756
Phone: (603) 650-7692
Fax: (603) 650-8086
Percentage of IMGs in the program: 10%
Minimum USMLE Step 1 Score Requirement: 206
Minimum USMLE Step 2 Score Requirement: 210
Attempts on any step: No limits set
CS required at time of application: No
USCE Requirement: None
Cut-Off time since graduation: No limits set
Program offers couple match: Yes
Visas Sponsored or accepted: J1 visa

New Jersey

Atlantic Health (Morristown) General Surgery Residency Program

Specialty: General Surgery
Program name: Atlantic Health (Morristown) Program
Program code: 440-33-11-183
NRMP Code: 1394440C0, 1394440P0
Program type: Community-based
State: New Jersey
Address: Morristown Medical Center
100 Madison Ave, Morristown, NJ 07962
Phone: (973) 971-5684
Fax: (973) 290-7350
Percentage of IMGs in the program: 40%
Minimum USMLE Step 1 Score Requirement: 220
Minimum USMLE Step 2 Score Requirement: 220
Attempts on any step: No limits set
CS required at time of application: Yes including ECFMG certificate
USCE Requirement: Yes
Cut-Off time since graduation: 5 years
Program offers couple match: Yes
Visas Sponsored or accepted: J1 visa

Cooper Medical School of Rowan University/Cooper University Hospital General Surgery Residency Program

Specialty: General Surgery
Program name: Cooper Medical School of Rowan University/Cooper University Hospital Program
Program code: 440-33-21-179
NRMP Code: 1380440C0
Program type: University-based
State: New Jersey
Address: Cooper Hospital-University Medical Center
                3 Cooper Plaza, Camden, NJ 08103
Phone: (856) 342-3012
Fax: (856) 365-7582
Percentage of IMGs in the program: 0%
Minimum USMLE Step 1 Score Requirement: 215
Minimum USMLE Step 2 Score Requirement: 210
Attempts on any step: Must pass on the first attempt
CS required at time of application: Yes including ECFMG certificate
USCE Requirement: None
Cut-Off time since graduation: 2 years

Program offers couple match: Yes
Visas Sponsored or accepted: No visa

Monmouth Medical Center General Surgery Residency Program

Specialty: General Surgery
Program name: Monmouth Medical Center Program
Program code: 440-33-21-182
NRMP Code: 1392440P0, 1392440C0
Program type: Community-based university affiliated hospital
State: New Jersey
Address: Monmouth Medical Center
300 Second Ave, Long Branch, NJ 07740
Phone: (732) 923-6769
Fax: (732) 923-6768
Percentage of IMGs in the program: 70%
Minimum USMLE Step 1 Score Requirement: 200
Minimum USMLE Step 2 Score Requirement: 210
Attempts on any step: Must pass on the first attempt
CS required at time of application: Yes including ECFMG certificate
USCE Requirement: Yes, 12 months
Cut-Off time since graduation: 3 years

Program offers couple match: Yes
Visas Sponsored or accepted: No visa

Rutgers New Jersey Medical School General Surgery Residency Program

Specialty: General Surgery
Program name: Rutgers New Jersey Medical School Program
Program code: 440-33-21-184
NRMP Code: 1398440P2, 1398440C0, 1398440P0
Program type: University-based
State: New Jersey
Address: Rutgers New Jersey Medical School
              185 S Orange Ave, Newark, NJ 07103
Phone: (973) 972-5682
Fax: (973) 972-6591
Percentage of IMGs in the program: 10% (Prelim IMGs only)
Minimum USMLE Step 1 Score Requirement: No limits set
Minimum USMLE Step 2 Score Requirement: No limits set
Attempts on any step: No limits set
CS required at time of application: Yes including ECFMG certificate
USCE Requirement: None
Cut-Off time since graduation: 5 years

Program offers couple match: Yes
Visas Sponsored or accepted: J1 visa

Rutgers Robert Wood Johnson Medical School General Surgery Residency Program

Specialty: General Surgery
Program name: Rutgers Robert Wood Johnson Medical School Program
Program code: 440-33-21-187
NRMP Code: 2918440C0, 2918440P0
Program type: University-based
State: New Jersey
Address: Rutgers Robert Wood Johnson Medical School
          51 French St, New Brunswick, NJ 08903-0019
Phone: (732) 235-7674
Fax: (732) 235-8372
Percentage of IMGs in the program: 20%
Minimum USMLE Step 1 Score Requirement: 220
Minimum USMLE Step 2 Score Requirement: 220
Attempts on any step: No limits set
CS required at time of application: Yes including ECFMG certificate
USCE Requirement: None
Cut-Off time since graduation: No limits set

Program offers couple match: Yes
Visas Sponsored or accepted: No visa

St Barnabas Medical Center General Surgery Residency Program

Specialty: General Surgery
Program name: St Barnabas Medical Center Program
Program code: 440-33-22-181
NRMP Code: 1396440P0, 1396440C0
Program type: Community-based university affiliated hospital
State: New Jersey
Address: St Barnabas Medical Center
            94 Old Short Hills Rd, Livingston, NJ 07039
Phone: (973) 322-8945
Fax: (973) 322-2471
Percentage of IMGs in the program: 40%
Minimum USMLE Step 1 Score Requirement: 220
Minimum USMLE Step 2 Score Requirement: 220
Attempts on any step: Must pass on the first attempt
CS required at time of application: Yes including ECFMG certificate
USCE Requirement: Yes, 12 months preferred
Cut-Off time since graduation: 5 years

Program offers couple match: Yes
Visas Sponsored or accepted: J1 visa

New Mexico

University of New Mexico General Surgery Residency Program

Specialty: General Surgery
Program name: University of New Mexico Program
Program code: 440-34-21-190
NRMP Code: 1962440C0, 1962440P0, 1962440P1
Program type: University-based
State: New Mexico
Address: University of New Mexico Health Science Center
        1 University of New Mexico, Albuquerque, NM 87131-0001
Phone: (505) 272-4161
Fax: (505) 272-8145
Percentage of IMGs in the program: 20%
Minimum USMLE Step 1 Score Requirement: 230
Minimum USMLE Step 2 Score Requirement: 230

Attempts on any step: Must pass on the first attempt
CS required at time of application: Yes including ECFMG certificate
USCE Requirement: None
Cut-Off time since graduation: 2 years
Program offers couple match: Yes
Visas Sponsored or accepted: J1 visa

New York

New York Medical College at Metropolitan Hospital Center General Surgery Residency Program

Specialty: General Surgery
Program name: New York Medical College at Metropolitan Hospital Center Program
Program code: 440-35-00-438
NRMP Code: 1473440C0, 1473440P0
Program type: Community-based university affiliated hospital

State: New York
Address: Metropolitan Hospital Center
          1901 First Ave, New York, NY 10029
Phone: (212) 423-6058
Fax: (212) 423-8002
Percentage of IMGs in the program: 60%
Minimum USMLE Step 1 Score Requirement:
220
Minimum USMLE Step 2 Score Requirement:
220
Attempts on any step: No limits set
CS required at time of application: Yes
including ECFMG certificate
USCE Requirement: Yes
Cut-Off time since graduation: No limits set
Program offers couple match: Yes
Visas Sponsored or accepted: J1 visa

Lincoln Medical and Mental Health Center General Surgery Residency Program

Specialty: General Surgery
Program name: Lincoln Medical and Mental Health Center Program
Program code: 440-35-00-439
NRMP Code: 1484440C0
Program type: Community-based university affiliated hospital
State: New York

Address: Lincoln Medical and Mental Health Center

  234 E 149th St, Bronx, NY 10451

Phone: (718) 579-5900   Ext: 5725
Fax: (718) 579-4620
Percentage of IMGs in the program: 70%
Minimum USMLE Step 1 Score Requirement: 220
Minimum USMLE Step 2 Score Requirement: 220
Attempts on any step: No limits set
CS required at time of application: Yes including ECFMG certificate
USCE Requirement: None
Cut-Off time since graduation: No limits set
Program offers couple match: Yes
Visas Sponsored or accepted: J1 visa and H1b visa

Icahn School of Medicine at Mount Sinai (Beth Israel) General Surgery Residency Program

Specialty: General Surgery
Program name: Icahn School of Medicine at Mount Sinai (Beth Israel) Program
Program code: 440-35-11-204
State: New York
Address: Icahn School of Medicine Mount Sinai Beth Israel

First Ave at 16th St, New York, NY 10003
Phone: (212) 420-4340
Fax: (212) 844-1939
Percentage of IMGs in the program: 10%
Minimum USMLE Step 1 Score Requirement: 225
Minimum USMLE Step 2 Score Requirement: 225
Attempts on any step: Must pass on first attempt
CS required at time of application: No
USCE Requirement: Yes
Cut-Off time since graduation: No limits set
Program offers couple match: Yes
Visas Sponsored or accepted: J1 visa

New York Hospital Medical Center of Queens/Cornell University Medical College General Surgery Residency Program

Specialty: General Surgery
Program name: New York Hospital Medical Center of Queens/Cornell University Medical College Program
Program code: 440-35-11-205
NRMP Code: 1822440P0, 1822440C0
Program type: Community-based university affiliated hospital

State: New York
Address: New York Hosp Queens
          56-45 Main St, Flushing, NY 11355
Phone: (718) 670-1572
Fax: (718) 670-1864
Percentage of IMGs in the program: 20%
Minimum USMLE Step 1 Score Requirement: 215
Minimum USMLE Step 2 Score Requirement: 215
Attempts on any step: Must pass on first attempt
CS required at time of application: No
USCE Requirement: None
Cut-Off time since graduation: 5 years
Program offers couple match: No
Visas Sponsored or accepted: J1 visa and H1b visa

Bronx-Lebanon Hospital Center General Surgery Residency Program

Specialty: General Surgery
Program name: Bronx-Lebanon Hospital Center Program
Program code: 440-35-11-206
NRMP Code: 1471440P0, 1471440C0
Program type: Community-based university affiliated hospital

State: New York
Address: Bronx-Lebanon Hospital Center
            1650 Selwyn Ave, Bronx, NY 10457
Phone: (718) 960-1216
Fax: (718) 960-1370
Percentage of IMGs in the program: 90%
Minimum USMLE Step 1 Score Requirement: 220
Minimum USMLE Step 2 Score Requirement: 220
Attempts on any step: Must pass on first attempt
CS required at time of application: Yes including ECFMG certificate
USCE Requirement: None
Cut-Off time since graduation: 8 years
Program offers couple match: Yes
Visas Sponsored or accepted: J1 visa and H1b visa

Harlem Hospital Center General Surgery Residency Program

Specialty: General Surgery
Program name: Harlem Hospital Center Program
Program code: 440-35-11-214
NRMP Code: 1478440P0, 1478440C0
Program type: Community-based
State: New York

Address: Harlem Hospital Center
             506 Lenox Ave, New York, NY 10037
Phone: (212) 939-1641
Fax: (212) 939-3599
Percentage of IMGs in the program: 100%
Minimum USMLE Step 1 Score Requirement: 230
Minimum USMLE Step 2 Score Requirement: 230
Attempts on any step: Must pass maximum on the 2nd attempt
CS required at time of application: Yes including ECFMG certificate
USCE Requirement: None
Cut-Off time since graduation: 5 years
Program offers couple match: No
Visas Sponsored or accepted: J1 visa and H1b visa

NSLIJ/Hofstra North Shore-LIJ School of Medicine at Lenox Hill Hospital General Surgery Residency Program

Specialty: General Surgery
Program name: NSLIJ/Hofstra North Shore-LIJ School of Medicine at Lenox Hill Hospital Program
Program code: 440-35-11-217
State: New York

Address: NS-LIJ Lenox Hill Hospital
            100 E 77th St, New York, NY 10075
Phone: (212) 434-2150
Fax: (212) 434-2083
Percentage of IMGs in the program: 50%
Minimum USMLE Step 1 Score Requirement: 215
Minimum USMLE Step 2 Score Requirement: 215
Attempts on any step: Must pass on the first attempt
CS required at time of application: Yes including ECFMG certificate
USCE Requirement: None
Cut-Off time since graduation: 3 years
Program offers couple match: Yes
Visas Sponsored or accepted: J1 visa and H1b visa

Staten Island University Hospital General Surgery Residency Program

Specialty: General Surgery
Program name: Staten Island University Hospital Program
Program code: 440-35-11-236
State: New York

Address: Staten Island University Hospital
475 Seaview Ave, Staten Island, NY 10305
Phone: (718) 226-1873
Fax: (718) 226-8395
Percentage of IMGs in the program: 60%
Minimum USMLE Step 1 Score Requirement: No limits set
Minimum USMLE Step 2 Score Requirement: No limits set
Attempts on any step: No limits set
CS required at time of application: No
USCE Requirement: None
Cut-Off time since graduation: No limits set
Program offers couple match: Yes
Visas Sponsored or accepted: H1b visa

Nassau University Medical Center General Surgery Residency Program

Specialty: General Surgery
Program name: Nassau University Medical Center Program
Program code: 440-35-12-198
NRMP Code: 1448440C0, 1448440P0
Program type: Community-based university affiliated hospital
State: New York

Address: Nassau University Medical Center
2201 Hempstead Trnpk, East Meadow, NY 11554
Phone: (516) 296-3389
Fax: (516) 572-5140
Percentage of IMGs in the program: 50%
Minimum USMLE Step 1 Score Requirement: No limits set
Minimum USMLE Step 2 Score Requirement: No limits set
Attempts on any step: No limits set
CS required at time of application: Yes including ECFMG certificate
USCE Requirement: None
Cut-Off time since graduation: 5 years
Program offers couple match: Yes
Visas Sponsored or accepted: J1 visa

NSLIJHS/Hofstra North Shore-LIJ School of Medicine General Surgery Residency Program

Specialty: General Surgery
Program name: NSLIJHS/Hofstra North Shore-LIJ School of Medicine Program
Program code: 440-35-13-411
NRMP Code: 1700440P0, 1700440C0, 1700440P1
Program type: University-based
State: New York

Address: Hofstra North Shore LIJ School of Medicine

270-05 76th Ave, New Hyde Park, NY 11040

Phone: (718) 470-4475
Fax: (718) 962-2239
Percentage of IMGs in the program: 30%
Minimum USMLE Step 1 Score Requirement: 205
Minimum USMLE Step 2 Score Requirement: 205
Attempts on any step: Must pass on first attempt
CS required at time of application: No
USCE Requirement: None
Cut-Off time since graduation: 3 years
Program offers couple match: No
Visas Sponsored or accepted: J1 visa and H1b visa

Albany Medical Center General Surgery Residency Program

Specialty: General Surgery
Program name: Albany Medical Center Program
Program code: 440-35-21-191
NRMP Code: 1414440P0, 1414440C0
Program type: University-based
State: New York

Address: Albany Medical Center
47 New Scotland Ave, Albany, NY 12208
Phone: (518) 262-5374
Fax: (518) 262-6397
Percentage of IMGs in the program: 15%
Minimum USMLE Step 1 Score Requirement: 210
Minimum USMLE Step 2 Score Requirement: 210
Attempts on any step: No limits set
CS required at time of application: Yes including ECFMG certificate
USCE Requirement: Yes, 12 months
Cut-Off time since graduation: 3 years
Program offers couple match: Yes
Visas Sponsored or accepted: No visa

Albert Einstein College of Medicine General Surgery Residency Program

Specialty: General Surgery
Program name: Albert Einstein College of Medicine Program
Program code: 440-35-21-202
NRMP Code: 3153440P3, 3153440C0, 3153440P1, 3153440P2
Program type: University-based
State: New York

Address: Montefiore Medical Center
3400 Bainbridge Ave, Bronx, NY 10467
Phone: (718) 696-2583
Fax: (718) 881-5074
Percentage of IMGs in the program: 25%
Minimum USMLE Step 1 Score Requirement: 225
Minimum USMLE Step 2 Score Requirement: 225
Attempts on any step: Must pass on the first attempt
CS required at time of application: No
USCE Requirement: Yes, 12 months
Cut-Off time since graduation: No limits set
Program offers couple match: Yes
Visas Sponsored or accepted: J1 visa and H1b visa

Brookdale University Hospital and Medical Center General Surgery Residency Program

Specialty: General Surgery
Program name: Brookdale University Hospital and Medical Center Program
Program code: 440-35-21-207
State: New York
Address: Brookdale University Hospital and Medical Center

One Brookdale Plaza, Brooklyn, NY 11212
Phone: (718) 240-6386
Percentage of IMGs in the program: 40%
Minimum USMLE Step 1 Score Requirement: 210
Minimum USMLE Step 2 Score Requirement: 210
Attempts on any step: No limits set
CS required at time of application: No
USCE Requirement: None
Cut-Off time since graduation: 5 years
Program offers couple match: Yes
Visas Sponsored or accepted: J1 visa and H1b visa

New York Presbyterian Hospital (Cornell Campus) General Surgery Residency Program

Specialty: General Surgery
Program name: New York Presbyterian Hospital (Cornell Campus) Program
Program code: 440-35-21-211
State: New York
Address: New York Presbyterian Hospital-Cornell
525 E 68th St, New York, NY 10065
Phone: (212) 746-5380
Fax: (212) 746-8802

Percentage of IMGs in the program: 20%
Minimum USMLE Step 1 Score Requirement: 220
Minimum USMLE Step 2 Score Requirement: 220
Attempts on any step: No limits set
CS required at time of application: No
USCE Requirement: None
Cut-Off time since graduation: No limits set
Program offers couple match: Yes
Visas Sponsored or accepted: J1 visa

Maimonides Medical Center General Surgery Residency Program

Specialty: General Surgery
Program name: Maimonides Medical Center Program
Program code: 440-35-21-221
NRMP Code:
Program type:
State: New York
Address: Maimonides Medical Center
4802 Tenth Ave, Brooklyn, NY 11219
Phone: (718) 283-7683
Fax: (718) 635-7157
Percentage of IMGs in the program: 50%
Minimum USMLE Step 1 Score Requirement: 220

Minimum USMLE Step 2 Score Requirement:
220
Attempts on any step: Must pass on first attempt
CS required at time of application: No
USCE Requirement: None
Cut-Off time since graduation: No limits set
Program offers couple match: Yes
Visas Sponsored or accepted: J1 visa and H1b visa

New York Methodist Hospital General Surgery Residency Program

Specialty: General Surgery
Program name: New York Methodist Hospital Program
Program code: 440-35-21-222
NRMP Code: 1429440C0, 1429440P0
Program type: Community-based university affiliated hospital
State: New York
Address: New York Methodist Hospital
          506 6th St, Brooklyn, NY 11215
Phone: (718) 780-7106
Fax: (718) 780-3154
Percentage of IMGs in the program: 50%
Minimum USMLE Step 1 Score Requirement:
220

Minimum USMLE Step 2 Score Requirement: 220
Attempts on any step: Must pass on the first attempt
CS required at time of application: No
USCE Requirement: None
Cut-Off time since graduation: No limits set
Program offers couple match: Yes
Visas Sponsored or accepted: No visa

Icahn School of Medicine at Mount Sinai General Surgery Residency Program

Specialty: General Surgery
Program name: Icahn School of Medicine at Mount Sinai Program
Program code: 440-35-21-225
State: New York
Address: Mount Sinai School of Medicine
5 E 98th St, New York, NY 10029
Phone: (212) 241-5967
Fax: (212) 410-0111
Percentage of IMGs in the program: 0%
Minimum USMLE Step 1 Score Requirement: No limits set
Minimum USMLE Step 2 Score Requirement: No limits set
Attempts on any step: No limits set
CS required at time of application: No

USCE Requirement: None
Cut-Off time since graduation: 5 years
Program offers couple match: Yes
Visas Sponsored or accepted: J1 visa and H1b visa

New York Medical College at Westchester Medical Center General Surgery Residency Program

Specialty: General Surgery
Program name: New York Medical College at Westchester Medical Center Program
Program code: 440-35-21-227
NRMP Code: 2998440C0, 2998440P0
Program type: University-based
State: New York
Address: NYMC Westchester Medical Center
        Taylor Pavilion Room E173, Valhalla, NY 10595
Phone: (914) 493-7614
Fax: (914) 493-1679
Percentage of IMGs in the program: 50%
Minimum USMLE Step 1 Score Requirement: 205
Minimum USMLE Step 2 Score Requirement: 220
Attempts on any step: Must pass on first attempt

CS required at time of application: Yes including ECFMG certificate
USCE Requirement: None
Cut-Off time since graduation: No limits set
Program offers couple match: Yes
Visas Sponsored or accepted: No visa

New York Presbyterian Hospital (Columbia Campus) General Surgery Residency Program

Specialty: General Surgery
Program name: New York Presbyterian Hospital (Columbia Campus) Program
Program code: 440-35-21-229
NRMP Code: 1495440P2, 1495440P0, 1495440C0
Program type: University-based
State: New York
Address: New York Presbyterian Hospital-Columbia
177 Fort Washington Ave, New York, NY 10032
Phone: (212) 305-3038
Fax: (212) 305-8321
Percentage of IMGs in the program: 10%
Minimum USMLE Step 1 Score Requirement: 236
Minimum USMLE Step 2 Score Requirement: 236

Attempts on any step: Must pass on first attempt
CS required at time of application: Yes including ECFMG certificate
USCE Requirement: None
Cut-Off time since graduation: No limits set
Program offers couple match: Yes
Visas Sponsored or accepted: J1 visa

SUNY Health Science Center at Brooklyn General Surgery Residency Program

Specialty: General Surgery
Program name: SUNY Health Science Center at Brooklyn Program
Program code: 440-35-21-237
NRMP Code: 1426440C0, 1426440P0,
Program type: University-based
State: New York
Address: SUNY Downstate Medical Center
450 Clarkson Ave, Brooklyn, NY 11203
Phone: (718) 270-3302
Fax: (718) 270-4676
Percentage of IMGs in the program: 20%
Minimum USMLE Step 1 Score Requirement: No limits set
Minimum USMLE Step 2 Score Requirement: No limits set
Attempts on any step: No limits set

CS required at time of application: Yes including ECFMG certificate
USCE Requirement: None
Cut-Off time since graduation: No limits set
Program offers couple match: Yes
Visas Sponsored or accepted: J1 visa

University of Rochester General Surgery Residency Program

Specialty: General Surgery
Program name: University of Rochester Program
Program code: 440-35-21-240
NRMP Code: 1511440C0, 1511440P0, 1511440P2
Program type: University-based
State: New York
Address: University of Rochester Medical Center
          601 Elmwood Ave, Rochester, NY 14642-8410
Phone: (585) 275-2723
Fax: (585) 276-2504
Percentage of IMGs in the program: 15%
Minimum USMLE Step 1 Score Requirement: No limits set
Minimum USMLE Step 2 Score Requirement: No limits set
Attempts on any step: No limits set

CS required at time of application: No
USCE Requirement: None
Cut-Off time since graduation: No limits set
Program offers couple match: Yes
Visas Sponsored or accepted: J1 visa

SUNY at Stony Brook General Surgery Residency Program

Specialty: General Surgery
Program name: SUNY at Stony Brook Program
Program code: 440-35-21-242
NRMP Code: 2919440P1, 2919440C0, 2919440P0,
Program type: University-based
State: New York
Address: SUNY Stony Brook University
         90 Nicolls Rd, Stony Brook, NY 11794-8191
Phone: (631) 444-1791
Fax: (631) 444-7689
Percentage of IMGs in the program: 10%
Minimum USMLE Step 1 Score Requirement: 230
Minimum USMLE Step 2 Score Requirement: 230
Attempts on any step: Must pass on the first attempt
CS required at time of application: Yes including ECFMG certificate

USCE Requirement: None
Cut-Off time since graduation: 3 years
Program offers couple match: Yes
Visas Sponsored or accepted: J1 visa

SUNY Upstate Medical University General Surgery Residency Program

Specialty: General Surgery
Program name: SUNY Upstate Medical University Program
Program code: 440-35-21-244
State: New York
Address: SUNY Upstate Medical University
750 E Adams St, Syracuse, NY 13210
Phone: (315) 464-6289
Percentage of IMGs in the program: 20%
Minimum USMLE Step 1 Score Requirement: 225
Minimum USMLE Step 2 Score Requirement: 225
Attempts on any step: Must pass on the first attempt
CS required at time of application: Yes including ECFMG certificate if already graduated
USCE Requirement: Yes
Cut-Off time since graduation: 5 years
Program offers couple match: Yes
Visas Sponsored or accepted: J1 visa

Icahn School of Medicine at Mount Sinai/St Luke's-Roosevelt Hospital Center General Surgery Residency Program

Specialty: General Surgery
Program name: Icahn School of Medicine at Mount Sinai/St Luke's-Roosevelt Hospital Center Program
Program code: 440-35-21-383
State: New York
Address: St Luke's-Roosevelt Hospital Center
1000 Tenth Ave, New York, NY 10019
Phone: (212) 523-6970
Fax: (212) 523-6495
Percentage of IMGs in the program: 15%
Minimum USMLE Step 1 Score Requirement: 235
Minimum USMLE Step 2 Score Requirement: 235
Attempts on any step: No limits set
CS required at time of application: Yes including ECFMG certificate
USCE Requirement: None
Cut-Off time since graduation: No limits set
Program offers couple match: Yes
Visas Sponsored or accepted: J1 visa and H1b visa

University at Buffalo General Surgery Residency Program

Specialty: General Surgery
Program name: University at Buffalo Program
Program code: 440-35-21-393
State: New York
Address: Buffalo General Medical Center
             100 High St, Buffalo, NY 14203
Phone: (716) 859-2810
Fax: (716) 859-7760
Percentage of IMGs in the program: 20%
Minimum USMLE Step 1 Score Requirement: No limits set
Minimum USMLE Step 2 Score Requirement: No limits set
Attempts on any step: No limits set
CS required at time of application: Yes including ECFMG certificate
USCE Requirement: None
Cut-Off time since graduation: No limits set
Program offers couple match: Yes
Visas Sponsored or accepted: J1 visa

New York University School of Medicine General Surgery Residency Program

Specialty: General Surgery

Program name: New York University School of Medicine Program
Program code: 440-35-21-394
NRMP Code: 2978440P0, 2978440P1, 2978440C0
Program type: University-based
State: New York
Address: New York University Medical Center
    550 First Ave, New York, NY 10016
Phone: (212) 263-6378
Fax: (212) 263-8216
Percentage of IMGs in the program: 0%
Minimum USMLE Step 1 Score Requirement: No limits set
Minimum USMLE Step 2 Score Requirement: No limits set
Attempts on any step: No limits set
CS required at time of application: Yes including ECFMG certificate
USCE Requirement: None
Cut-Off time since graduation: No limits set
Program offers couple match: Yes
Visas Sponsored or accepted: J1 visa and H1b visa

Bassett Medical Center General Surgery Residency Program

Specialty: General Surgery

Program name: Bassett Medical Center Program
Program code: 440-35-31-197
NRMP Code: 1442440P0, 1442440C0
Program type: Community-based university affiliated hospital
State: New York
Address: Bassett Medical Centre
            One Atwell Rd, Cooperstown, NY 13326
Phone: (888) 547-6349
Fax: (607) 547-6553
Percentage of IMGs in the program: 0%
Minimum USMLE Step 1 Score Requirement: No limits set
Minimum USMLE Step 2 Score Requirement: No limits set
Attempts on any step: Must pass on the first attempt
CS required at time of application: Yes including ECFMG certificate
USCE Requirement: None
Cut-Off time since graduation: No limits set
Program offers couple match: Yes
Visas Sponsored or accepted: J1 visa

Brooklyn Hospital Center General Surgery Residency Program

Specialty: General Surgery

Program name: Brooklyn Hospital Center Program
Program code: 440-35-31-208
NRMP Code: 1420440C0
Program type: Community-based university affiliated hospital
State: New York
Address: Brooklyn Hospital Center
 121 DeKalb Ave, Brooklyn, NY 11201
Phone: (718) 250-6923
Fax: (718) 250-8919
Percentage of IMGs in the program: 80%
Minimum USMLE Step 1 Score Requirement: 230
Minimum USMLE Step 2 Score Requirement: 230
Attempts on any step: Must pass on the first attempt
CS required at time of application: Yes including ECFMG certificate
USCE Requirement: None
Cut-Off time since graduation: No limits set
Program offers couple match: Yes
Visas Sponsored or accepted: J1 visa

North Carolina

Vidant Medical Center/East Carolina University General Surgery Residency Program

Specialty: General Surgery
Program name: Vidant Medical Center/East Carolina University Program
Program code: 440-36-11-248
State: North Carolina
Address: Brody School of Medicine ECU
       600 Moye Blvd, Greenville, NC 27834
Phone: (252) 744-5069
Fax: (252) 744-3156
Percentage of IMGs in the program: 0%
Minimum USMLE Step 1 Score Requirement: 230
Minimum USMLE Step 2 Score Requirement: 230
Attempts on any step: No limits set
CS required at time of application: Yes including ECFMG certificate
USCE Requirement: None
Cut-Off time since graduation: No limits set
Program offers couple match: Yes
Visas Sponsored or accepted: J1 visa

Carolinas Medical Center General Surgery Residency Program

Specialty: General Surgery
Program name: Carolinas Medical Center Program
Program code: 440-36-12-246
NRMP Code: 1527440C0, 1527440P0
Program type: Community-based university affiliated hospital
State: North Carolina
Address: Carolinas Medical Center
　　　　　1000 Blythe Blvd, Charlotte, NC 28232-2861
Phone: (704) 355-3641
Fax: (704) 355-5619
Percentage of IMGs in the program: 10%
Minimum USMLE Step 1 Score Requirement: No limits set
Minimum USMLE Step 2 Score Requirement: No limits set
Attempts on any step: No limits set
CS required at time of application: Yes including ECFMG certificate
USCE Requirement: None
Cut-Off time since graduation: No limits set
Program offers couple match: Yes
Visas Sponsored or accepted: No visa

University of North Carolina Hospitals General Surgery Residency Program

Specialty: General Surgery
Program name: University of North Carolina Hospitals Program
Program code: 440-36-21-245
NRMP Code: 1900440P0, 1900440C0
Program type: University-based
State: North Carolina
Address: University of North Carolina Hospitals
101 Manning Dr, Chapel Hill, NC 27599-7050
Phone: (919) 966-4653
Fax: (919) 966-7841
Percentage of IMGs in the program: 5%
Minimum USMLE Step 1 Score Requirement: No limits set
Minimum USMLE Step 2 Score Requirement: No limits set
Attempts on any step: No limits set
CS required at time of application: No
USCE Requirement: None
Cut-Off time since graduation: No limits set
Program offers couple match: Yes
Visas Sponsored or accepted: J1 visa

Duke University Hospital General Surgery Residency Program

Specialty: General Surgery
Program name: Duke University Hospital Program

Program code: 440-36-21-247
NRMP Code: 1529440P3, 1529440C0
Program type: University-based
State: North Carolina
Address: Duke University Medical Center
           200 Tent Drive, Durham, NC 27710
Phone: (919) 681-3816
Fax: (919) 681-8856
Percentage of IMGs in the program: 5% (Prelim mostly)
Minimum USMLE Step 1 Score Requirement: No limits set
Minimum USMLE Step 2 Score Requirement: No limits set
Attempts on any step: No limits set
CS required at time of application: Yes including ECFMG certificate
USCE Requirement: None
Cut-Off time since graduation: No limits set
Program offers couple match: Yes
Visas Sponsored or accepted: J1 visa

New Hanover Regional Medical Center General Surgery Residency Program

Specialty: General Surgery
Program name: New Hanover Regional Medical Center Program
Program code: 440-36-31-249

NRMP Code: 1534440P0, 1534440C0
Program type: Community-based university affiliated hospital
State: North Carolina
Address: New Hanover Regional Medical Center
2131 S 17th St, Wilmington, NC 28402
Phone: (910) 667-9287
Fax: (910) 763-4630
Percentage of IMGs in the program: 0%
Minimum USMLE Step 1 Score Requirement: 205
Minimum USMLE Step 2 Score Requirement: 205
Attempts on any step: Must pass on the first attempt
CS required at time of application: Yes including ECFMG certificate
USCE Requirement: 2 years
Cut-Off time since graduation: 2 years
Program offers couple match: Yes
Visas Sponsored or accepted: No visa

Wake Forest University School of Medicine General Surgery Residency Program

Specialty: General Surgery
Program name: Wake Forest University School of Medicine Program
Program code: 440-36-31-250

NRMP Code: 1537440P0, 1537440C0
Program type: University-based
State: North Carolina
Address: Wake Forest Baptist Medical Center
Medical Center Blvd, Winston-Salem,
NC 27157
Phone: (336) 716-7496
Fax: (336) 716-5414
Percentage of IMGs in the program: 5%
Minimum USMLE Step 1 Score Requirement:
230
Minimum USMLE Step 2 Score Requirement:
230
Attempts on any step: No limits set
CS required at time of application: Yes
including ECFMG certificate
USCE Requirement: Yes
Cut-Off time since graduation: No limits set
Program offers couple match: Yes
Visas Sponsored or accepted: J1 visa

North Dakota

University of North Dakota General Surgery Residency Program

Specialty: General Surgery

Program name: University of North Dakota Program
Program code: 440-37-21-379
NRMP Code: 1539440C0, 1539440P0, 1539440C1
Program type: Community-based university affiliated hospital
State: North Dakota
Address: University of North Dakota
501 N Columbia Rd, Grand Forks, ND 58202-9037
Phone: (701) 777-3067
Fax: (701) 777-2609
Percentage of IMGs in the program: 0%
Minimum USMLE Step 1 Score Requirement: 210
Minimum USMLE Step 2 Score Requirement: 210
Attempts on any step: Must pass on the first attempt
CS required at time of application: Yes including ECFMG certificate
USCE Requirement: 3 months
Cut-Off time since graduation: No limits set, but prefer within 5 years
Program offers couple match: Yes
Visas Sponsored or accepted: J1 visa

Ohio

Akron General Medical Center/NEOMED General Surgery Residency Program

Specialty: General Surgery
Program name: Akron General Medical Center/NEOMED Program
Program code: 440-38-11-252
NRMP Code: 1542440P2, 1542440C0
Program type: Community-based university affiliated hospital
State: Ohio
Address: Akron General Medical Center
          1 Akron General Ave, Akron, OH 44307
Phone: (330) 344-6741
Fax: (330) 344-6672
Percentage of IMGs in the program: 0%
Minimum USMLE Step 1 Score Requirement: 230
Minimum USMLE Step 2 Score Requirement: 230
Attempts on any step: Must pass on the first attempt
CS required at time of application: Yes including ECFMG certificate
USCE Requirement: None
Cut-Off time since graduation: 5 years
Program offers couple match: Yes

Visas Sponsored or accepted: J1 visa and H1b visa

St Elizabeth Health Center/NEOMED General Surgery Residency Program

Specialty: General Surgery
Program name: St Elizabeth Health Center/NEOMED Program
Program code: 440-38-11-270
NRMP Code: 1584440C0
Program type: Community-based university affiliated hospital
State: Ohio
Address: St Elizabeth Health Center
1044 Belmont Ave, Youngstown, OH 44501-1790
Phone: (330) 480-3124
Fax: (330) 480-3640
Percentage of IMGs in the program: 50%
Minimum USMLE Step 1 Score Requirement: 220
Minimum USMLE Step 2 Score Requirement: 220
Attempts on any step: No limits set
CS required at time of application: Yes including ECFMG certificate
USCE Requirement: None
Cut-Off time since graduation: 3 years

Program offers couple match: Yes
Visas Sponsored or accepted: J1 visa

Riverside Methodist Hospitals (OhioHealth) General Surgery Residency Program

Specialty: General Surgery
Program name: Riverside Methodist Hospitals (OhioHealth) Program
Program code: 440-38-12-265
NRMP Code: 1567440P0, 1567440C0
Program type: Community-based
State: Ohio
Address: Riverside Methodist Hospital
3535 Olentangy River Rd, Columbus, OH 43214
Phone: (614) 566-5468
Fax: (614) 566-1073
Percentage of IMGs in the program: 10%
Minimum USMLE Step 1 Score Requirement: 210
Minimum USMLE Step 2 Score Requirement: 210
Attempts on any step: No limits set
CS required at time of application: Yes including ECFMG certificate
USCE Requirement: None
Cut-Off time since graduation: No limits set
Program offers couple match: Yes

Visas Sponsored or accepted: J1 visa

Summa Health System/NEOMED General Surgery Residency Program

Specialty: General Surgery
Program name: Summa Health System/NEOMED Program
Program code: 440-38-21-251
NRMP Code: 1541440C0, 1541440P0
Program type: Community-based
State: Ohio
Address: Summa Health System
       55 Arch St, Akron, OH 44304
Phone: (330) 375-6299
Fax: (330) 375-3751
Percentage of IMGs in the program: 0%
Minimum USMLE Step 1 Score Requirement: 210
Minimum USMLE Step 2 Score Requirement: 210
Attempts on any step: No limits set
CS required at time of application: No
USCE Requirement: None
Cut-Off time since graduation: 4 years
Program offers couple match: Yes
Visas Sponsored or accepted: J1 visa

University of Cincinnati Medical Center/College of Medicine General Surgery Residency Program

Specialty: General Surgery
Program name: University of Cincinnati Medical Center/College of Medicine Program
Program code: 440-38-21-255
NRMP Code: 1548440C0, 1548440P0
Program type: University-based
State: Ohio
Address: University of Cincinnati Medical Center
231 Albert Sabin Way, Cincinnati, OH 45267-0558
Phone: (513) 558-4206
Fax: (513) 558-3474
Percentage of IMGs in the program: 0%
Minimum USMLE Step 1 Score Requirement: 230
Minimum USMLE Step 2 Score Requirement: 230
Attempts on any step: No limits set
CS required at time of application: No
USCE Requirement: None
Cut-Off time since graduation: No limits set
Program offers couple match: Yes
Visas Sponsored or accepted: No visa

Ohio State University Hospital General Surgery Residency Program

Specialty: General Surgery
Program name: Ohio State University Hospital Program
Program code: 440-38-21-264
NRMP Code: 1566440C0, 1566440P0, 1566440P1
Program type: University-based
State: Ohio
Address: Ohio State University Wexner Medical Center
         395 W 12th Ave, Columbus, OH 43210-1250
Phone: (614) 293-8704
Fax: (614) 293-4063
Percentage of IMGs in the program: 0%
Minimum USMLE Step 1 Score Requirement: 215
Minimum USMLE Step 2 Score Requirement: 215
Attempts on any step: No limits set
CS required at time of application: Yes including ECFMG certificate
USCE Requirement: Yes, 1 year
Cut-Off time since graduation: No limits set
Program offers couple match: Yes
Visas Sponsored or accepted: J1 visa

Wright State University General Surgery Residency Program

Specialty: General Surgery
Program name: Wright State University Program
Program code: 440-38-21-266
NRMP Code: 2011440P0, 2011440C0
Program type: Community-based university affiliated hospital
State: Ohio
Address: Miami Valley Hospital
         128 E Apple St, Dayton, OH 45409-2793
Phone: (937) 208-2485
Fax: (937) 208-2105
Percentage of IMGs in the program: 5%
Minimum USMLE Step 1 Score Requirement: 225
Minimum USMLE Step 2 Score Requirement: 225
Attempts on any step: Must pass maximum from the 2nd attempt
CS required at time of application: Yes including ECFMG certificate
USCE Requirement: None
Cut-Off time since graduation: 2 years
Program offers couple match: Yes
Visas Sponsored or accepted: No visa

University of Toledo General Surgery Residency Program

Specialty: General Surgery
Program name: University of Toledo Program
Program code: 440-38-21-269
NRMP Code: 1579440C0, 1579440P0, 1579440P1
Program type: University-based
State: Ohio
Address: University of Toledo Medical Center
3000 Arlington Ave, Toledo, OH 43614-2598
Phone: (419) 383-6462
Fax: (419) 383-3348
Percentage of IMGs in the program: 40%
Minimum USMLE Step 1 Score Requirement: 210
Minimum USMLE Step 2 Score Requirement: 210
Attempts on any step: Must pass on the first attempt
CS required at time of application: Yes including ECFMG certificate
USCE Requirement: None
Cut-Off time since graduation: No limits set
Program offers couple match: Yes
Visas Sponsored or accepted: J1 visa

Western Reserve Health Education/NEOMED General Surgery Residency Program

Specialty: General Surgery
Program name: Western Reserve Health Education/NEOMED Program
Program code: 440-38-21-271
NRMP Code: 1585440C0, 1585440P0
Program type: Community-based university affiliated hospital
State: Ohio
Address: Northside Medical Center
500 Gypsy Ln, Youngstown, OH 44501-0990
Phone: (330) 884-3815
Fax: (330) 884-5730
Percentage of IMGs in the program: 50%
Minimum USMLE Step 1 Score Requirement: 220
Minimum USMLE Step 2 Score Requirement: 220
Attempts on any step: Must pass on the first attempt
CS required at time of application: Yes including ECFMG certificate
USCE Requirement: Yes
Cut-Off time since graduation: 2 years
Program offers couple match: Yes
Visas Sponsored or accepted: J1 visa case by case only

Case Western Reserve University/University Hospitals Case Medical Center General Surgery Residency Program

Specialty: General Surgery
Program name: Case Western Reserve University/University Hospitals Case Medical Center Program
Program code: 440-38-21-399
NRMP Code: 1552440C0, 1552440P2, 1552440P0
Program type: University-based
State: Ohio
Address: University Hospitals Case Medical Center
11100 Euclid Ave, Cleveland, OH 44106
Phone: (216) 844-3027
Fax: (216) 844-2888
Percentage of IMGs in the program: 20% (Mainly Prelims)
Minimum USMLE Step 1 Score Requirement: 230
Minimum USMLE Step 2 Score Requirement: 230
Attempts on any step: Must pass on first attempt
CS required at time of application: Yes

including ECFMG certificate
USCE Requirement: Yes with US LORs
Cut-Off time since graduation: 2 years
Program offers couple match: No
Visas Sponsored or accepted: J1 visa

Cleveland Clinic Foundation General Surgery Residency Program

Specialty: General Surgery
Program name: Cleveland Clinic Foundation Program
Program code: 440-38-22-257
NRMP Code: 1968440P0, 1968440C0
Program type: Community-based university affiliated hospital
State: Ohio
Address: Cleveland Clinic
9500 Euclid Ave, Cleveland, OH 44195
Phone: (216) 444-2009
Fax: (216) 444-1162
Percentage of IMGs in the program: 15%
Minimum USMLE Step 1 Score Requirement: No limits set
Minimum USMLE Step 2 Score Requirement: No limits set
Attempts on any step: No limits set
CS required at time of application: Yes including ECFMG certificate

USCE Requirement: None
Cut-Off time since graduation: No limits set
Program offers couple match: Yes
Visas Sponsored or accepted: J1 visa and H1b visa

TriHealth (Good Samaritan Hospital) General Surgery Residency Program

Specialty: General Surgery
Program name: TriHealth (Good Samaritan Hospital) Program
Program code: 440-38-31-253
State: Ohio
Address: Good Samaritan Hospital
375 Dixmyth Ave, Cincinnati, OH 45220
Phone: (513) 862-3562
Fax: (513) 221-5865
Percentage of IMGs in the program: 10%
Minimum USMLE Step 1 Score Requirement: 210
Minimum USMLE Step 2 Score Requirement: 210
Attempts on any step: No limits set
CS required at time of application: Yes including ECFMG certificate
USCE Requirement: Yes, 3 months
Cut-Off time since graduation: 1 year

Program offers couple match: Yes
Visas Sponsored or accepted: J1 visa

Jewish Hospital of Cincinnati General Surgery Residency Program

Specialty: General Surgery
Program name: Jewish Hospital of Cincinnati Program
Program code: 440-38-31-254
NRMP Code: 1551440P0, 1551440C0
Program type: Community-based university affiliated hospital
State: Ohio
Address: The Jewish Hospital of Cincinnati
4777 E Galbraith Rd, Cincinnati, OH 45236
Phone: (513) 686-5466
Fax: (513) 686-5469
Percentage of IMGs in the program: 60%
Minimum USMLE Step 1 Score Requirement: 215
Minimum USMLE Step 2 Score Requirement: 215
Attempts on any step: Must pass on the first attempt
CS required at time of application: Yes including ECFMG certificate
USCE Requirement: Yes

Cut-Off time since graduation: 2 years
Program offers couple match: Yes
Visas Sponsored or accepted: J1 visa

Mount Carmel Health System General Surgery Residency Program

Specialty: General Surgery
Program name: Mount Carmel Health System Program
Program code: 440-38-32-263
State: Ohio
Address: Mount Carmel-West Hospital
793 W State St, Columbus, OH 43222
Phone: (614) 234-5983
Fax: (614) 234-2772
Percentage of IMGs in the program: 0%
Minimum USMLE Step 1 Score Requirement: 210
Minimum USMLE Step 2 Score Requirement: 210
Attempts on any step: Must pass on the first attempt
CS required at time of application: Yes including ECFMG certificate
USCE Requirement: Yes
Cut-Off time since graduation: Must be in final year
Program offers couple match: Yes

Visas Sponsored or accepted: No visa

Oklahoma

University of Oklahoma Health Sciences Center General Surgery Residency Program

Specialty: General Surgery
Program name: University of Oklahoma Health Sciences Center Program
Program code: 440-39-21-273
NRMP Code: 1588440P3, 1588440C0, 1588440P4
Program type: University-based
State: Oklahoma
Address: University of Oklahoma Health Sciences Center
          PO Box 26901, Oklahoma City, OK 73126
Phone: (405) 271-6308
Fax: (405) 271-3919
Percentage of IMGs in the program: 20%
Minimum USMLE Step 1 Score Requirement: 210
Minimum USMLE Step 2 Score Requirement: 210

Attempts on any step: No limits set
CS required at time of application: No
USCE Requirement: None
Cut-Off time since graduation: No limits set
Program offers couple match: Yes
Visas Sponsored or accepted: J1 visa

University of Oklahoma School of Community Medicine (Tulsa) General Surgery Residency Program

Specialty: General Surgery
Program name: University of Oklahoma School of Community Medicine (Tulsa) Program
Program code: 440-39-21-274
NRMP Code: 2727440P0, 2727440C0
Program type: University-based
State: Oklahoma
Address: University of Oklahoma School of Community Medicine
      4502 E 41st St, Tulsa, OK 74135-2512
Phone: (918) 634-7539
Fax: (918) 634-7567
Percentage of IMGs in the program: 10%
Minimum USMLE Step 1 Score Requirement: 220
Minimum USMLE Step 2 Score Requirement: 220

Attempts on any step: Must pass on the maximum the 3rd attempt on any step
CS required at time of application: Yes including ECFMG certificate
USCE Requirement: Yes
Cut-Off time since graduation: 3 years
Program offers couple match: Yes
Visas Sponsored or accepted: J1 visa and H1b visa for select cases

Oregon

Oregon Health & Science University General Surgery Residency Program

Specialty: General Surgery
Program name: Oregon Health & Science University Program
Program code: 440-40-21-278
NRMP Code: 1599440C0, 1599440P0
Program type: University-based
State: Oregon
Address: Oregon Health & Science University
          3181 SW Sam Jackson Park Rd,
Portland, OR 97239-3098

Phone: (503) 494-4936
Fax: (503) 494-5615
Percentage of IMGs in the program: 0%
Minimum USMLE Step 1 Score Requirement: 210
Minimum USMLE Step 2 Score Requirement: 210
Attempts on any step: Must pass on the first attempt
CS required at time of application: Yes including ECFMG certificate
USCE Requirement: None
Cut-Off time since graduation: No limits set
Program offers couple match: Yes
Visas Sponsored or accepted: No visa

Pennsylvania

Conemaugh Valley Memorial Hospital General Surgery Residency Program

Specialty: General Surgery
Program name: Conemaugh Valley Memorial Hospital Program
Program code: 440-41-11-288
NRMP Code: 1616440P0, 1616440C0

Program type: Community-based university affiliated hospital
State: Pennsylvania
Address: Conemaugh Memorial Medical Center 1086 Franklin St, Johnstown, PA 15905
Phone: (814) 534-1660
Fax: (814) 534-1680
Percentage of IMGs in the program: 30%
Minimum USMLE Step 1 Score Requirement: 220
Minimum USMLE Step 2 Score Requirement: 220
Attempts on any step: No limits set
CS required at time of application: Yes including ECFMG certificate
USCE Requirement: None
Cut-Off time since graduation: 4 years
Program offers couple match: Yes
Visas Sponsored or accepted: J1 visa

Albert Einstein Healthcare Network General Surgery Residency Program

Specialty: General Surgery
Program name: Albert Einstein Healthcare Network Program
Program code: 440-41-11-291

NRMP Code: 1631440C0, 1631440P0, 1631440R0
Program type: Community-based university affiliated hospital
State: Pennsylvania
Address: Albert Einstein Medical Center
5501 Old York Rd, Philadelphia, PA 19141
Phone: (215) 456-3443
Fax: (215) 456-3529
Percentage of IMGs in the program: 20%
Minimum USMLE Step 1 Score Requirement: No limits set
Minimum USMLE Step 2 Score Requirement: No limits set
Attempts on any step: No limits set
CS required at time of application: Yes including ECFMG certificate
USCE Requirement: None
Cut-Off time since graduation: No limits set
Program offers couple match: Yes
Visas Sponsored or accepted: J1 visa

Main Line Health System/Lankenau Medical Center General Surgery Residency Program

Specialty: General Surgery
Program name: Main Line Health System/Lankenau Medical Center Program

Program code: 440-41-11-296
NRMP Code: 1632440C0
Program type: Community-based university affiliated hospital
State: Pennsylvania
Address: Lankenau Medical Center
100 Lancaster Ave, Wynnewood, PA 19096
Phone: (484) 476-2164
Fax: (484) 476-3354
Percentage of IMGs in the program: 40%
Minimum USMLE Step 1 Score Requirement: 220
Minimum USMLE Step 2 Score Requirement: 220
Attempts on any step: Must pass on the first attempt on any step
CS required at time of application: Yes including ECFMG certificate
USCE Requirement: 6 months
Cut-Off time since graduation: 3 years
Program offers couple match: Yes
Visas Sponsored or accepted: J1 visa and H1b visa

Abington Memorial Hospital General Surgery Residency Program

Specialty: General Surgery

Program name: Abington Memorial Hospital Program
Program code: 440-41-12-279
NRMP Code: 1600440C0, 1600440P0
Program type: Community-based university affiliated hospital
State: Pennsylvania
Address: Abington Memorial Hospital
            1200 Old York Rd, Abington, PA 19001
Phone: (215) 481-7320
Fax: (215) 481-2159
Percentage of IMGs in the program: 20% (variable)
Minimum USMLE Step 1 Score Requirement: 220
Minimum USMLE Step 2 Score Requirement: 220
Attempts on any step: Must pass on the first attempt
CS required at time of application: Yes including ECFMG certificate
USCE Requirement: None
Cut-Off time since graduation: No limits set
Program offers couple match: Yes
Visas Sponsored or accepted: J1 visa

Allegheny General Hospital-Western Pennsylvania Hospital Medical Education Consortium (AGH) General Surgery Residency Program

Specialty: General Surgery
Program name: Allegheny General Hospital-Western Pennsylvania Hospital Medical Education Consortium (AGH) Program
Program code: 440-41-12-303
NRMP Code: 1648440P0, 1648440C0
Program type: Community-based university affiliated hospital
State: Pennsylvania
Address: Allegheny General Hospital
320 E North Ave, Pittsburgh, PA 15212-9986
Phone: (412) 359-6907
Fax: (412) 359-3212
Percentage of IMGs in the program: 5%
Minimum USMLE Step 1 Score Requirement: No limits set
Minimum USMLE Step 2 Score Requirement: No limits set
Attempts on any step: No limits set
CS required at time of application: No
USCE Requirement: Yes with 2 US LORs
Cut-Off time since graduation: No limits set
Program offers couple match: Yes

Visas Sponsored or accepted: J1 visa

UPMC Medical Education (Mercy) General Surgery Residency Program

Specialty: General Surgery
Program name: UPMC Medical Education (Mercy) Program
Program code: 440-41-12-305
State: Pennsylvania
Address: UPMC Mercy
    1400 Locust St, Pittsburgh, PA 15219
Phone: (412) 232-5528
Fax: (412) 232-8096
Percentage of IMGs in the program: 20%
Minimum USMLE Step 1 Score Requirement: 220
Minimum USMLE Step 2 Score Requirement: 220
Attempts on any step: No limits set
CS required at time of application: No
USCE Requirement: Yes, 1 month
Cut-Off time since graduation: 5 years
Program offers couple match: Yes
Visas Sponsored or accepted: J1 visa

Robert Packer Hospital/Guthrie General Surgery Residency Program

Specialty: General Surgery
Program name: Robert Packer Hospital/Guthrie Program
Program code: 440-41-12-309
NRMP Code: 1664440P0, 1664440C0
Program type: Community-based university affiliated hospital
State: Pennsylvania
Address: Guthrie/Robert Packer Hospital
One Guthrie Sq, Sayre, PA 18840-1698
Phone: (570) 887-3585
Fax: (570) 887-3599
Percentage of IMGs in the program: 15%
Minimum USMLE Step 1 Score Requirement: 210
Minimum USMLE Step 2 Score Requirement: 210
Attempts on any step: Must pass on the first attempt
CS required at time of application: Yes including ECFMG certificate
USCE Requirement: None but 1 month preferred
Cut-Off time since graduation: 3 years
Program offers couple match: Yes

Visas Sponsored or accepted: J1 visa and H1b visa

York Hospital General Surgery Residency Program

Specialty: General Surgery
Program name: York Hospital Program
Program code: 440-41-12-310
NRMP Code: 1674440P0, 1674440C0
Program type: Community-based university affiliated hospital
State: Pennsylvania
Address: York Hospital
         1001 S George St, York, PA 17405
Phone: (717) 851-4362
Fax: (717) 851-4513
Percentage of IMGs in the program: 20% (Variable)
Minimum USMLE Step 1 Score Requirement: 210
Minimum USMLE Step 2 Score Requirement: 210
Attempts on any step: Must pass on the first attempt
CS required at time of application: Yes including ECFMG certificate at time of ranking
USCE Requirement: None
Cut-Off time since graduation: 5 years
Program offers couple match: Yes

Visas Sponsored or accepted: J1 visa and H1b visa

Lehigh Valley Health Network/University of South Florida College of Medicine General Surgery Residency Program

Specialty: General Surgery
Program name: Lehigh Valley Health Network/University of South Florida College of Medicine Program
Program code: 440-41-21-280
NRMP Code: 1601440C0, 1601440P1
Program type: Community-based university affiliated hospital
State: Pennsylvania
Address: Lehigh Valley Health Network
         Cedar Crest & I-78, Allentown, PA 18105-1556
Phone: (610) 402-8966
Fax: (610) 402-1667
Percentage of IMGs in the program: 0%
Minimum USMLE Step 1 Score Requirement: 220
Minimum USMLE Step 2 Score Requirement: 220
Attempts on any step: Must pass on the first attempt
CS required at time of application: No

USCE Requirement: None
Cut-Off time since graduation: No limits set
Program offers couple match: Yes
Visas Sponsored or accepted: No

Geisinger Health System General Surgery Residency Program

Specialty: General Surgery
Program name: Geisinger Health System Program
Program code: 440-41-21-283
State: Pennsylvania
Address: Geisinger Medical Center
        100 N Academy Ave, Danville, PA 17822-2169
Phone: (570) 271-5900
Fax: (570) 271-8324
Percentage of IMGs in the program: 40%
Minimum USMLE Step 1 Score Requirement: No limits set
Minimum USMLE Step 2 Score Requirement: No limits set
Attempts on any step: Must pass on the first attempt
CS required at time of application: Yes including ECFMG certificate
USCE Requirement: None
Cut-Off time since graduation: No limits set
Program offers couple match: Yes

Visas Sponsored or accepted: J1 visa

Penn State Milton S Hershey Medical Center General Surgery Residency Program

Specialty: General Surgery
Program name: Penn State Milton S Hershey Medical Center Program
Program code: 440-41-21-287
NRMP Code: 1617440P0, 1617440P1, 1617440C0
Program type: University-based
State: Pennsylvania
Address: Penn State Milton S Hershey Medical Center
500 University Dr, Hershey, PA 17033-0850
Phone: (717) 531-8557
Fax: (717) 531-5393
Percentage of IMGs in the program: 0%
Minimum USMLE Step 1 Score Requirement: No limits set
Minimum USMLE Step 2 Score Requirement: No limits set
Attempts on any step: No limits set
CS required at time of application: No
USCE Requirement: None
Cut-Off time since graduation: No limits set

Program offers couple match: Yes
Visas Sponsored or accepted: J1 visa

Drexel University College of Medicine/Hahnemann University Hospital General Surgery Residency Program

Specialty: General Surgery
Program name: Drexel University College of Medicine/Hahnemann University Hospital Program
Program code: 440-41-21-295
NRMP Code: 1849440P0, 1849440C0
Program type: University-based
State: Pennsylvania
Address: Hahnemann University Hospital
245 N 15th St, Philadelphia, PA 19102
Phone: (215) 762-3585
Fax: (215) 762-3058
Percentage of IMGs in the program: 30%
Minimum USMLE Step 1 Score Requirement: 220
Minimum USMLE Step 2 Score Requirement: 220
Attempts on any step: Must pass on the first attempt
CS required at time of application: No
USCE Requirement: None
Cut-Off time since graduation: 5 years

Program offers couple match: Yes
Visas Sponsored or accepted: J1 visa

Temple University Hospital General Surgery Residency Program

Specialty: General Surgery
Program name: Temple University Hospital Program
Program code: 440-41-21-300
Program type: University based
State: Pennsylvania
Address: Temple University Hospital
3401 N Broad St, Philadelphia, PA 19140
Phone: (215) 707-3632
Fax: 215-707-1915
Percentage of IMGs in the program: 30%
Minimum USMLE Step 1 Score Requirement: 225
Minimum USMLE Step 2 Score Requirement: 225
Attempts on any step: Must pass on the first attempt
CS required at time of application: Yes including ECFMG certificate
USCE Requirement: None
Cut-Off time since graduation: No limits set
Program offers couple match: Yes

Visas Sponsored or accepted: J1 visa and H1b visa

Thomas Jefferson University General Surgery Residency Program

Specialty: General Surgery
Program name: Thomas Jefferson University Program
Program code: 440-41-21-301
NRMP Code: 1630440C0, 1630440P0
Program type: University-based
State: Pennsylvania
Address: Thomas Jefferson University Hospital
      1015 Walnut St, Philadelphia, PA 19107
Phone: (215) 955-6864
Fax: (215) 955-2878
Percentage of IMGs in the program: 5%
Minimum USMLE Step 1 Score Requirement: 230
Minimum USMLE Step 2 Score Requirement: 230
Attempts on any step: Must pass on
CS required at time of application: Yes including ECFMG certificate
USCE Requirement: None
Cut-Off time since graduation: No limits set
Program offers couple match: Yes

Visas Sponsored or accepted: J1 visa and H1b visa

University of Pennsylvania General Surgery Residency Program

Specialty: General Surgery
Program name: University of Pennsylvania Program
Program code: 440-41-21-302
NRMP Code: 1628440P3, 1628440P0, 1628440C0, 1628440P1
Program type: University-based
State: Pennsylvania
Address: Hospital of University of Pennsylvania
3400 Spruce St, Philadelphia, PA 19104
Phone: (215) 662-6156
Fax: (215) 662-7983
Percentage of IMGs in the program: 10% (Variable, mostly prelims)
Minimum USMLE Step 1 Score Requirement: No limits set
Minimum USMLE Step 2 Score Requirement: No limits set
Attempts on any step: No limits set
CS required at time of application: Yes including ECFMG certificate
USCE Requirement: None
Cut-Off time since graduation: 10 years

Program offers couple match: Yes
Visas Sponsored or accepted: J1 visa

UPMC Medical Education General Surgery Residency Program

Specialty: General Surgery
Program name: UPMC Medical Education Program
Program code: 440-41-21-304
State: Pennsylvania
Address: University of Pittsburgh Medical Center
           200 Lothrop St, Pittsburgh, PA 15213
Phone: (412) 647-3389
Fax: (412) 647-1999
Percentage of IMGs in the program: 15%
Minimum USMLE Step 1 Score Requirement: No limits set
Minimum USMLE Step 2 Score Requirement: No limits set
Attempts on any step: No limits set
CS required at time of application: Yes including ECFMG certificate
USCE Requirement: None
Cut-Off time since graduation: No limits set
Program offers couple match: Yes
Visas Sponsored or accepted: J1 visa

PinnacleHealth Hospitals General Surgery Residency Program

Specialty: General Surgery
Program name: PinnacleHealth Hospitals Program
Program code: 440-41-21-384
State: Pennsylvania
Address: PinnacleHealth System
          205 S Front St, Harrisburg, PA 17104
Phone: (717) 231-8755
Fax: (717) 231-8756
Percentage of IMGs in the program: 40%
Minimum USMLE Step 1 Score Requirement: 220
Minimum USMLE Step 2 Score Requirement: 220
Attempts on any step: Must pass on first attempt
CS required at time of application: Yes including ECFMG certificate
USCE Requirement: Yes, 1 year
Cut-Off time since graduation: 5 years
Program offers couple match: Yes
Visas Sponsored or accepted: No visa

St Luke's Hospital General Surgery Residency Program

Specialty: General Surgery
Program name: St Luke's Hospital Program
Program code: 440-41-21-398
NRMP Code: 1605440C0
Program type: University-based
State: Pennsylvania
Address: St Luke's University Hospital
          801 Ostrum St, Bethlehem, PA 18015
Phone: (484) 526-2255
Fax: (484) 526-2217
Percentage of IMGs in the program: 30%
Minimum USMLE Step 1 Score Requirement:
No limits set
Minimum USMLE Step 2 Score Requirement:
No limits set
Attempts on any step: No limits set
CS required at time of application: No
USCE Requirement: None
Cut-Off time since graduation: No limits set
Program offers couple match: No
Visas Sponsored or accepted: J1 visa

Easton Hospital General Surgery Residency Program

Specialty: General Surgery
Program name: Easton Hospital Program
Program code: 440-41-31-284
NRMP Code: 1610440C0, 1610440P0
Program type: Community-based university

affiliated hospital
State: Pennsylvania
Address: Easton Hospital
        250 South 21st St, Easton, PA 18042
Phone: (610) 250-4375
Fax: (610) 250-4851
Percentage of IMGs in the program: 70%
Minimum USMLE Step 1 Score Requirement: 210
Minimum USMLE Step 2 Score Requirement: 210
Attempts on any step: Must pass on the first attempt
CS required at time of application: Yes including ECFMG certificate
USCE Requirement: None but helpful
Cut-Off time since graduation: 5 years
Program offers couple match: Yes
Visas Sponsored or accepted: J1 visa

Mercy Catholic Medical Center General Surgery Residency Program

Specialty: General Surgery
Program name: Mercy Catholic Medical Center Program
Program code: 440-41-31-297
NRMP Code: 1636440C0, 1636440P0
Program type: Community-based university

affiliated hospital
State: Pennsylvania
Address: Mercy Catholic Medical Center
         1500 Lansdowne Ave, Darby, PA 19023
Phone: (610) 237-4950
Fax: (610) 237-4329
Percentage of IMGs in the program: 50%
Minimum USMLE Step 1 Score Requirement: 210
Minimum USMLE Step 2 Score Requirement: 210
Attempts on any step: Must pass on the first attempt
CS required at time of application: Yes including ECFMG certificate
USCE Requirement: None
Cut-Off time since graduation: 5 years
Program offers couple match: Yes
Visas Sponsored or accepted: J1 visa and H1b visa

Rhode Island

Brown University General Surgery Residency Program

Specialty: General Surgery
Program name: Brown University Program
Program code: 440-43-21-314
NRMP Code: 1677440P0, 1677440C0
Program type: University-based
State: Rhode Island
Address: Rhode Island Hospital
593 Eddy St, Providence, RI 02903
Phone: (401) 444-5180
Fax: (401) 444-6681
Percentage of IMGs in the program: 10%
Minimum USMLE Step 1 Score Requirement: 225
Minimum USMLE Step 2 Score Requirement: 225
Attempts on any step: Must pass on the first attempt
CS required at time of application: No
USCE Requirement: 6 months
Cut-Off time since graduation: 5 years
Program offers couple match: Yes
Visas Sponsored or accepted: J1 visa

South Carolina

Grand Strand Regional Medical Center General Surgery Residency Program

Specialty: General Surgery
Program name: Grand Strand Regional Medical Center Program
Program code: 440-45-00-319
NRMP Code: 1761440C0, 1761440P0
Program type: Community-based university affiliated hospital
State: South Carolina
Address: Grand Strand Medical Center
          809 82nd Pkwy, Myrtle Beach, SC 29572
Phone: (843) 692-1595
Fax: (843) 692-1122
Percentage of IMGs in the program: 20%
Minimum USMLE Step 1 Score Requirement: 210
Minimum USMLE Step 2 Score Requirement: 210
Attempts on any step: Must pass on the first attempt
CS required at time of application: Yes including ECFMG certificate
USCE Requirement: None
Cut-Off time since graduation: 5 years, unless in residency or military service
Program offers couple match: Yes

Visas Sponsored or accepted: J1 visa

Greenville Health System/University of South Carolina General Surgery Residency Program

Specialty: General Surgery
Program name: Greenville Health System/University of South Carolina Program
Program code: 440-45-11-317
NRMP Code: 1683440C0, 1683440P0
Program type: Community-based university affiliated hospital
State: South Carolina
Address: Greenville Hospital System
701 Grove Rd, Greenville, SC 29605
Phone: (864) 455-1435
Fax: (864) 455-1320
Percentage of IMGs in the program: 20%
Minimum USMLE Step 1 Score Requirement: 225
Minimum USMLE Step 2 Score Requirement: 225
Attempts on any step: Must pass on the first attempt
CS required at time of application: Yes including ECFMG certificate
USCE Requirement: Yes
Cut-Off time since graduation: 2 years

Program offers couple match: Yes
Visas Sponsored or accepted: No visa

Medical University of South Carolina General Surgery Residency Program

Specialty: General Surgery
Program name: Medical University of South Carolina Program
Program code: 440-45-21-315
NRMP Code: 1680440C0, 1680440P0
Program type: University-based
State: South Carolina
Address: Medical University of South Carolina
         96 Jonathan Lucas St, Charleston, SC 29425
Phone: (843) 876-0179
Fax: (843) 792-4523
Percentage of IMGs in the program: 0%
Minimum USMLE Step 1 Score Requirement: 230
Minimum USMLE Step 2 Score Requirement: 230
Attempts on any step: Must pass on first attempt
CS required at time of application: Yes including ECFMG certificate
USCE Requirement: Yes
Cut-Off time since graduation: No limits set

Program offers couple match: Yes
Visas Sponsored or accepted: J1 visa

Palmetto Health/University of South Carolina School of Medicine General Surgery Residency Program

Specialty: General Surgery
Program name: Palmetto Health/University of South Carolina School of Medicine Program
Program code: 440-45-21-316
NRMP Code: 1681440C0, 1681440P0
Program type: Community-based university affiliated hospital
State: South Carolina
Address: USC Palmetto Health Richland
2 Richland Medical Pk, Columbia, SC 29203
Phone: (803) 545-5800
Fax: (803) 933-9545
Percentage of IMGs in the program: 30%
Minimum USMLE Step 1 Score Requirement: 210
Minimum USMLE Step 2 Score Requirement: 210
Attempts on any step: No limits set
CS required at time of application: No
USCE Requirement: None
Cut-Off time since graduation: No limits set

Program offers couple match: Yes
Visas Sponsored or accepted: No visa

Spartanburg Regional Healthcare System General Surgery Residency Program

Specialty: General Surgery
Program name: Spartanburg Regional Healthcare System Program
Program code: 440-45-31-318
State: South Carolina
Address: Spartanburg Regional Healthcare System
          101 E Wood St, Spartanburg, SC 29303
Phone: (864) 560-6285
Fax: (864) 560-6063
Percentage of IMGs in the program: 10%
Minimum USMLE Step 1 Score Requirement: No limits set
Minimum USMLE Step 2 Score Requirement: No limits set
Attempts on any step: No limits set
CS required at time of application: Yes including ECFMG certificate
USCE Requirement: Yes
Cut-Off time since graduation: 2 years
Program offers couple match: Yes

Visas Sponsored or accepted: No visa

South Dakota

University of South Dakota School of Medicine General Surgery Residency Program

Specialty: General Surgery
Program name: University of South Dakota School of Medicine Program
Program code: 440-46-00-001
State: South Dakota
Address: USD Sanford School of Medicine
1400 W 22nd St, Sioux Falls, SD 57105
Phone: (605) 357-1391
Fax: (605) 357-1528
Percentage of IMGs in the program: 20%
Minimum USMLE Step 1 Score Requirement: 220
Minimum USMLE Step 2 Score Requirement: 220
Attempts on any step: Must pas on the first attempt
CS required at time of application: No
USCE Requirement: Yes
Cut-Off time since graduation: 5 years unless clinically active

Program offers couple match: Yes
Visas Sponsored or accepted: J1 visa and H1b
visa

Tennessee

University of Tennessee College of Medicine at Chattanooga General Surgery Residency Program

Specialty: General Surgery
Program name: University of Tennessee College
of Medicine at Chattanooga Program
Program code: 440-47-11-320
NRMP Code: 1689440P0, 1689440C0
Program type: University-based
State: Tennessee
Address: University of Tennessee College of
Medicine-Chattanooga
            979 E Third St, Chattanooga, TN
37403
Phone: (423) 778-7695
Fax: (423) 778-2950
Percentage of IMGs in the program: 0%
Minimum USMLE Step 1 Score Requirement:
215

Minimum USMLE Step 2 Score Requirement: 215
Attempts on any step: Must pass on the first attempt
CS required at time of application: Yes including ECFMG certificate
USCE Requirement: 1-3 months with 3 US LORs
Cut-Off time since graduation: No limits set
Program offers couple match: Yes
Visas Sponsored or accepted: J1 visa

University of Tennessee Medical Center at Knoxville General Surgery Residency Program

Specialty: General Surgery
Program name: University of Tennessee Medical Center at Knoxville Program
Program code: 440-47-11-321
NRMP Code: 1839440C0, 1839440P0, 1839440P2
Program type: University-based
State: Tennessee
Address: University of Tennessee Memorial Hospital
       1924 Alcoa Hwy, Maryville, TN 37804
Phone: (865) 305-9230
Fax: (865) 305-8894
Percentage of IMGs in the program: 5%

Minimum USMLE Step 1 Score Requirement: No limits set

Minimum USMLE Step 2 Score Requirement: No limits set

Attempts on any step: Must pass on the first attempt

CS required at time of application: Yes including ECFMG certificate

USCE Requirement: Yes, 1 year

Cut-Off time since graduation: No limits set

Program offers couple match: Yes

Visas Sponsored or accepted: J1 visa

University of Tennessee General Surgery Residency Program

Specialty: General Surgery

Program name: University of Tennessee Program

Program code: 440-47-21-324

NRMP Code: 1844440C0, 1844440P0

Program type: University-based

State: Tennessee

Address: University of Tennessee Health Science Center

910 Madison Ave, Memphis, TN 38163

Phone: (901) 448-7635

Fax: (901) 448-7306

Percentage of IMGs in the program: 0%

Minimum USMLE Step 1 Score Requirement:
No limits set
Minimum USMLE Step 2 Score Requirement:
No limits set
Attempts on any step: No limits set
CS required at time of application: Yes
including ECFMG certificate
USCE Requirement: None
Cut-Off time since graduation: No limits set
Program offers couple match: Yes
Visas Sponsored or accepted: J1 visa

Vanderbilt University General Surgery Residency Program

Specialty: General Surgery
Program name: Vanderbilt University Program
Program code: 440-47-21-327
NRMP Code: 1702440C0, 1702440P0
Program type: University-based
State: Tennessee
Address: Vanderbilt University Medical Center
        1161 21st Ave S, Nashville, TN 37232-2730
Phone: (615) 343-6642
Fax: (615) 322-0689
Percentage of IMGs in the program: 0%
Minimum USMLE Step 1 Score Requirement:
No limits set

Minimum USMLE Step 2 Score Requirement: No limits set
Attempts on any step: No limits set
CS required at time of application: Yes including ECFMG certificate
USCE Requirement: None
Cut-Off time since graduation: No limits set
Program offers couple match: Yes
Visas Sponsored or accepted: J1 visa and H1b visa

East Tennessee State University General Surgery Residency Program

Specialty: General Surgery
Program name: East Tennessee State University Program
Program code: 440-47-21-377
NRMP Code: 2066440C0, 2066440P0
Program type: Community-based university affiliated hospital
State: Tennessee
Address: ETSU James H Quillen College of Medicine
         Box 70575, Johnson City, TN 37614
Phone: (423) 439-6267
Fax: (423) 439-6259
Percentage of IMGs in the program: 10%

Minimum USMLE Step 1 Score Requirement:
No limits set
Minimum USMLE Step 2 Score Requirement:
No limits set
Attempts on any step: No limits set
CS required at time of application: Yes
including ECFMG certificate
USCE Requirement: 1 year
Cut-Off time since graduation: 5 years
Program offers couple match: Yes
Visas Sponsored or accepted: J1 visa

Texas

University of Texas Health Science Center at San Antonio and Doctors Hospital at Renaissance (UT-Rio Grande Valley-Drs Hospital at Renaissance) General Surgery Residency Program

Specialty: General Surgery
Program name: University of Texas Health Science Center at San Antonio and Doctors Hospital at

Renaissance (UT-Rio Grande Valley-Drs Hospital at Renaissance) Program
Program code: 440-48-00-434
State: Texas
Address: Doctors Hospital at Renaissance
5321 S McColl Rd, Edinburg, TX 78539
Phone: (956) 362-3571
Fax: (956) 362-3599
Percentage of IMGs in the program: 15%
Minimum USMLE Step 1 Score Requirement: No limits set
Minimum USMLE Step 2 Score Requirement: No limits set
Attempts on any step: No limits set
CS required at time of application: Yes including ECFMG certificate
USCE Requirement: None
Cut-Off time since graduation: No limits set
Program offers couple match: Yes
Visas Sponsored or accepted: J1 visa

Texas Tech University Health Sciences Center Paul L Foster School of Medicine General Surgery Residency Program

Specialty: General Surgery
Program name: Texas Tech University Health Sciences Center Paul L Foster School of Medicine Program

Program code: 440-48-11-332
NRMP Code: 1710440C0, 1710440P0
Program type: University-based
State: Texas
Address: Texas Tech University HSC Paul L
Foster School of Medicine
            4800 Alberta Ave, El Paso, TX 79905
Phone: (915) 215-5310
Fax: (915) 545-6864
Percentage of IMGs in the program: 50%
Minimum USMLE Step 1 Score Requirement:
210
Minimum USMLE Step 2 Score Requirement:
210
Attempts on any step: Must pass on the first
attempt
CS required at time of application: Yes
including ECFMG certificate
USCE Requirement: None but might be
requested on their discretion
Cut-Off time since graduation: 5 years
Program offers couple match: Yes
Visas Sponsored or accepted: J1 visa

University of Texas Medical Branch Hospitals General Surgery Residency Program

Specialty: General Surgery

Program name: University of Texas Medical Branch Hospitals Program
Program code: 440-48-11-333
NRMP Code: 1714440C0, 1714440P0
Program type: University-based
State: Texas
Address: University of Texas Medical Branch Hospitals
       301 University Blvd, Galveston, TX 77555-0534
Phone: (409) 772-1369
Fax: (409) 772-0557
Percentage of IMGs in the program: 10%
Minimum USMLE Step 1 Score Requirement: No limits set
Minimum USMLE Step 2 Score Requirement: No limits set
Attempts on any step: No limits set
CS required at time of application: Yes including ECFMG certificate
USCE Requirement: None
Cut-Off time since graduation: No limits set
Program offers couple match: Yes
Visas Sponsored or accepted: J1 visa

Methodist Health System Dallas General Surgery Residency Program

Specialty: General Surgery

Program name: Methodist Health System Dallas Program
Program code: 440-48-12-329
NRMP Code: 1707440P0, 1707440C0
Program type: Community-based
State: Texas
Address: Methodist Health System Dallas
          1441 N Beckley Ave, Dallas, TX 75265-5999
Phone: (214) 947-2315
Fax: (214) 947-2361
Percentage of IMGs in the program: 15%
Minimum USMLE Step 1 Score Requirement: 210
Minimum USMLE Step 2 Score Requirement: 220
Attempts on any step: Must pass on the first attempt
CS required at time of application: Yes including ECFMG certificate
USCE Requirement: None
Cut-Off time since graduation: No limits set
Program offers couple match: Yes
Visas Sponsored or accepted: J1 visa

University of Texas at Austin Dell Medical School General Surgery Residency Program

Specialty: General Surgery

Program name: University of Texas at Austin Dell Medical School Program
Program code: 440-48-13-424
NRMP Code: 2835440C1
Program type: Community-based university affiliated hospital
State: Texas
Address: University Medical Center at Brackenridge
            601 E 15th St, Austin, TX 78701
Phone: (512) 324-7392
Fax: (512) 324-7399
Percentage of IMGs in the program: 0%
Minimum USMLE Step 1 Score Requirement: 220
Minimum USMLE Step 2 Score Requirement: 220
Attempts on any step: Must pass on the first attempt
CS required at time of application: Yes including ECFMG certificate
USCE Requirement: Yes, 1-2 month
Cut-Off time since graduation: 5 years
Program offers couple match: Yes
Visas Sponsored or accepted: J1 visa

Baylor University Medical Center General Surgery Residency Program

Specialty: General Surgery
Program name: Baylor University Medical Center Program
Program code: 440-48-21-328
NRMP Code: 1706440C0, 1706440P0
Program type: Community-based
State: Texas
Address: Baylor University Medical Center 3500 Gaston Ave, Dallas, TX 75246
Phone: (214) 820-4543
Fax: (214) 820-7272
Percentage of IMGs in the program: 0%
Minimum USMLE Step 1 Score Requirement: 220
Minimum USMLE Step 2 Score Requirement: 220
Attempts on any step: Must pass on the first attempt
CS required at time of application: No
USCE Requirement: None
Cut-Off time since graduation: 1 year
Program offers couple match: Yes
Visas Sponsored or accepted: J1 visa

University of Texas Southwestern Medical School General Surgery Residency Program

Specialty: General Surgery
Program name: University of Texas Southwestern Medical School Program
Program code: 440-48-21-331
NRMP Code: 2835440C0, 2835440P0, 2835440P2
Program type: University-based
State: Texas
Address: University of Texas Southwestern Medical Center
5323 Harry Hines Blvd, Dallas, TX 75390-9159
Phone: (214) 648-3515
Fax: (214) 648-6752
Percentage of IMGs in the program: 0%
Minimum USMLE Step 1 Score Requirement: 240
Minimum USMLE Step 2 Score Requirement: 240
Attempts on any step: Must pass on the first attempt
CS required at time of application: Yes including ECFMG certificate
USCE Requirement: None
Cut-Off time since graduation: 1 year
Program offers couple match: Yes
Visas Sponsored or accepted: J1 visa

Baylor College of Medicine General Surgery Residency Program

Specialty: General Surgery
Program name: Baylor College of Medicine Program
Program code: 440-48-21-334
NRMP Code: 1716440C0, 1716440C1, 1716440P0, 1716440P1
Program type: University-based
State: Texas
Address: Baylor College of Medicine
One Baylor Plaza, Houston, TX 77030
Phone: (713) 798-6078
Fax: (713) 798-8941
Percentage of IMGs in the program: 0%
Minimum USMLE Step 1 Score Requirement: No limits set
Minimum USMLE Step 2 Score Requirement: No limits set
Attempts on any step: No limits set
CS required at time of application: Yes including ECFMG certificate
USCE Requirement: None
Cut-Off time since graduation: No limits set
Program offers couple match: Yes
Visas Sponsored or accepted: J1 visa

University of Texas at Houston General Surgery Residency Program

Specialty: General Surgery
Program name: University of Texas at Houston Program
Program code: 440-48-21-337
State: Texas
Address: University of Texas Medical School at Houston
         6431 Fannin St, Houston, TX 77030
Phone: (713) 500-7216
Fax: (713) 486-0971
Percentage of IMGs in the program: 0%
Minimum USMLE Step 1 Score Requirement: 230
Minimum USMLE Step 2 Score Requirement: 230
Attempts on any step: No limits set
CS required at time of application: Yes including ECFMG certificate
USCE Requirement: None
Cut-Off time since graduation: No limits set
Program offers couple match: Yes
Visas Sponsored or accepted: J1 visa

University of Texas Health Science Center at San Antonio General Surgery Residency Program

Specialty: General Surgery
Program name: University of Texas Health Science Center at San Antonio Program
Program code: 440-48-21-338
NRMP Code: 1722440P0, 1722440C0, 1722440C1
Program type: University-based
State: Texas
Address: University of Texas HSC San Antonio
7703 Floyd Curl Dr, San Antonio, TX 78229-3900
Phone: (210) 567-5711
Percentage of IMGs in the program: 20%
Minimum USMLE Step 1 Score Requirement: 230
Minimum USMLE Step 2 Score Requirement: 230
Attempts on any step: Must pass on the first attempt
CS required at time of application: Yes including ECFMG certificate
USCE Requirement: None but highly desirable
Cut-Off time since graduation: No limits set
Program offers couple match: Yes
Visas Sponsored or accepted: J1 visa

Specialty: General Surgery
Program name: Texas A&M College of
Medicine-Scott and White Program
Program code: 440-48-21-339
NRMP Code: 1725440P1, 1725440C0,
1725440P0
Program type: University-based
State: Texas
Address: Scott and White Memorial
Hospital
            2401 S 31st St, Temple, TX
76508-0001
Phone: (254) 724-2366
Fax: (254) 724-7827
Percentage of IMGs in the program: 0%
**Minimum USMLE Step 1 Score
Requirement:** 220
**Minimum USMLE Step 2 Score
Requirement:** 220
Attempts on any step: Must pass on the
first attempt
CS required at time of application: Yes
including ECFMG certificate
USCE Requirement: None
Cut-Off time since graduation: No limits
set

Program offers couple match: Yes
Visas Sponsored or accepted: J1 visa

Texas Tech University (Lubbock) General Surgery Residency Program

Specialty: General Surgery
Program name: Texas Tech University (Lubbock) Program
Program code: 440-48-21-363
NRMP Code: 2973440C0, 2973440P0, 2973440P1
Program type: University-based
State: Texas
Address: Texas Tech University HSC Lubbock
        3601 4th St, Lubbock, TX 79430
Phone: (806) 743-3720
Fax: (806) 743-1475
Percentage of IMGs in the program: 30%
Minimum USMLE Step 1 Score Requirement: 220
Minimum USMLE Step 2 Score Requirement: 220
Attempts on any step: No limits set
CS required at time of application: No
USCE Requirement: None

Cut-Off time since graduation: No limits set
Program offers couple match: Yes
Visas Sponsored or accepted: J1 visa

Methodist Hospital (Houston) General Surgery Residency Program

Specialty: General Surgery
Program name: Methodist Hospital (Houston) Program
Program code: 440-48-22-335
State: Texas
Address: Houston Methodist Hospital
6550 Fannin St, Houston, TX 77030
Phone: (713) 441-6172
Fax: (713) 790-2872
Percentage of IMGs in the program: 20%
Minimum USMLE Step 1 Score Requirement: No limits set
Minimum USMLE Step 2 Score Requirement: No limits set
Attempts on any step: No limits set
CS required at time of application: Yes including ECFMG certificate
USCE Requirement: None
Cut-Off time since graduation: 3 years
Program offers couple match: Yes
Visas Sponsored or accepted: J1 visa

Utah

University of Utah General Surgery Residency Program

Specialty: General Surgery
Program name: University of Utah Program
Program code: 440-49-21-340
Program type: University-based
State: Utah
Address: University of Utah Medical Center
30 N 1900 E, Salt Lake City, UT 84132
Phone: (801) 581-6803
Fax: (801) 581-7122
Percentage of IMGs in the program: 10%
Minimum USMLE Step 1 Score Requirement: 220
Minimum USMLE Step 2 Score Requirement: 220
Attempts on any step: Must pass from first attempt
CS required at time of application: Yes including ECFMG certificate
USCE Requirement: Yes, 1year within the last 2 years
Cut-Off time since graduation: No limits set

Program offers couple match: Yes
Visas Sponsored or accepted: J1 visa

Vermont

University of Vermont Medical Center General Surgery Residency Program

Specialty: General Surgery
Program name: University of Vermont Medical Center Program
Program code: 440-50-21-341
Program type: University-based
State: Vermont
Address: University of Vermont Medical Center
111 Colchester Ave, Burlington, VT 05401
Phone: (802) 847-2566
Fax: (802) 847-9528
Percentage of IMGs in the program: 10%
Minimum USMLE Step 1 Score Requirement: No limits set
Minimum USMLE Step 2 Score Requirement: No limits set

Attempts on any step: No limits set
CS required at time of application: Yes including ECFMG certificate
USCE Requirement: Yes, within the past two years
Cut-Off time since graduation: 2 years
Program offers couple match: Yes
Visas Sponsored or accepted: J1 visa

Virginia

University of Virginia General Surgery Residency Program

Specialty: General Surgery
Program name: University of Virginia Program
Program code: 440-51-21-342
NRMP Code: 1737440C0, 1737440P0, 1737440P1
Program type: University-based
State: Virginia
Address: University of Virginia Health System
          Charlottesville, VA 22908-0681
Phone: (434)924-9307
Percentage of IMGs in the program: 5%

Minimum USMLE Step 1 Score Requirement:
210
Minimum USMLE Step 2 Score Requirement:
210
Attempts on any step: Must pass on the first attempt
CS required at time of application: Yes including ECFMG certificate
USCE Requirement: None
Cut-Off time since graduation: No limits set
Program offers couple match: No
Visas Sponsored or accepted: J1 visa

Eastern Virginia Medical School General Surgery Residency Program

Specialty: General Surgery
Program name: Eastern Virginia Medical School Program
Program code: 440-51-21-343
State: Virginia
Address: Eastern Virginia Medical School
825 Fairfax Ave, Norfolk, VA 23507-1912
Phone: (757) 446-8967
Fax: (757) 446-8407
Percentage of IMGs in the program: 0%
Minimum USMLE Step 1 Score Requirement:
No limits set

Minimum USMLE Step 2 Score Requirement: No limits set

Attempts on any step: No limits set

CS required at time of application: Yes including ECFMG certificate

USCE Requirement: Yes, 1-2 months

Cut-Off time since graduation: 2 years

Program offers couple match: Yes

Visas Sponsored or accepted: J1 visa

Virginia Commonwealth University Health System General Surgery Residency Program

Specialty: General Surgery

Program name: Virginia Commonwealth University Health System Program

Program code: 440-51-21-344

State: Virginia

Address: West Hospital Virginia Commonwealth University Health System
1200 E Broad St, Richmond, VA 23298-0135

Phone: (804) 828-2755

Fax: (804) 828-5595

Percentage of IMGs in the program: 0%

Minimum USMLE Step 1 Score Requirement: No limits set

Minimum USMLE Step 2 Score Requirement: No limits set

Attempts on any step: No limits set
CS required at time of application: No
USCE Requirement: Yes, 3 months
Cut-Off time since graduation: 4 years
Program offers couple match: Yes
Visas Sponsored or accepted: J1 visa

Inova Fairfax Medical Campus/Inova Fairfax Hospital for Children General Surgery Residency Program

Specialty: General Surgery
Program name: Inova Fairfax Medical Campus/Inova Fairfax Hospital for Children Program
Program code: 440-51-21-412
NRMP Code: 3199440C0
Program type: Community-based
State: Virginia
Address: Inova Fairfax Hospital
    3300 Gallows Rd, Falls Church, VA 22042
Phone: (703) 776-2337
Fax: (703) 776-2338
Percentage of IMGs in the program: 10%
Minimum USMLE Step 1 Score Requirement: 220
Minimum USMLE Step 2 Score

Requirement: 220
Attempts on any step: Must pass on the first attempt
CS required at time of application: No. If the ECFMG certificate obtained more than 18

months ago then TOEFL, TSE and TWE are required.
USCE Requirement: Yes, 3 months
Cut-Off time since graduation: 5 years or clinically active within the past 5 years.
Program offers couple match: Yes
Visas Sponsored or accepted: J1 visa and H1b visa

Carilion Clinic-Virginia Tech Carilion School of Medicine General Surgery Residency Program

Specialty: General Surgery
Program name: Carilion Clinic-Virginia Tech Carilion School of Medicine Program
Program code: 440-51-31-345
NRMP Code: 1748440P0, 1748440C0
Program type: Community-based university affiliated hospital
State: Virginia
Address: Carilion Roanoke Memorial Hospital
            1906 Belleview Ave SE, Roanoke, VA

24014
Phone: (540) 981-8280
Fax: (540) 981-8681
Percentage of IMGs in the program: 5%
Minimum USMLE Step 1 Score Requirement:
210
Minimum USMLE Step 2 Score Requirement:
210
Attempts on any step: No limits set
CS required at time of application: No
USCE Requirement: None
Cut-Off time since graduation: No limits set
Program offers couple match: Yes
Visas Sponsored or accepted: J1 visa

Washington

Virginia Mason Medical Center General Surgery Residency Program

Specialty: General Surgery
Program name: Virginia Mason Medical Center Program
Program code: 440-54-12-349
NRMP Code: 1756440P0, 1756440C0
Program type: Community-based

State: Washington
Address: Virginia Mason Medical Center
925 Seneca St, Seattle, WA 98111
Phone: (206) 341-1297
Fax: (206) 583-2307
Percentage of IMGs in the program: 0%
Minimum USMLE Step 1 Score Requirement: 210
Minimum USMLE Step 2 Score Requirement: 210
Attempts on any step: No limits set
CS required at time of application: Yes including ECFMG certificate
USCE Requirement: 6 months
Cut-Off time since graduation: 3 years unless you have USCE after graduation
Program offers couple match: Yes
Visas Sponsored or accepted: J1 visa

University of Washington General Surgery Residency Program

Specialty: General Surgery
Program name: University of Washington Program
Program code: 440-54-21-348
NRMP Code: 1918440P0, 1918440C0, 1918440P3
Program type: University-based
State: Washington

Address: University of Washington School of Medicine

       1959 NE Pacific St, Seattle, WA 98195-6410

Phone: (206) 543-3687

Fax: (206) 543-8136

Percentage of IMGs in the program: 0%

Minimum USMLE Step 1 Score Requirement: 220

Minimum USMLE Step 2 Score Requirement: 220

Attempts on any step: Must pass on the first attempt and within the last 3 years

CS required at time of application: Yes including ECFMG certificate

USCE Requirement: Must do this http://depts.washington.edu/uwsurgap/fmg.html

Cut-Off time since graduation: 10 years

Program offers couple match: Yes

Visas Sponsored or accepted: No visa

Swedish Medical Center/First Hill General Surgery Residency Program

Specialty: General Surgery

Program name: Swedish Medical Center/First Hill Program

Program code: 440-54-32-347

NRMP Code: 1755440P0, 1755440C0
Program type: Community-based
State: Washington
Address: Swedish Medical Center-First Hill
         747 Broadway, Seattle, WA 98122
Phone: (206) 386-2123
Fax: (206) 215-1521
Percentage of IMGs in the program: 0%
Minimum USMLE Step 1 Score Requirement: 230
Minimum USMLE Step 2 Score Requirement: 230
Attempts on any step: Must pass on the first attempt
CS required at time of application: No
USCE Requirement: Yes
Cut-Off time since graduation: 5 years
Program offers couple match: No
Visas Sponsored or accepted: No visa

West Virginia

Specialty: General Surgery
Program name: Charleston Area Medical
Center/West Virginia University (Charleston
Division) Program
Program code: 440-55-11-351
NRMP Code: 1902440P0, 1902440C0
Program type: Community-based
university affiliated hospital
State: West Virginia
Address: Charleston Area Medical Center
3110 MacCorkle Ave SE,
Charleston, WV 25304
Phone: (304) 347-1338
Fax: (304) 388-9958
Percentage of IMGs in the program: 10%
**Minimum USMLE Step 1 Score
Requirement:** 210
**Minimum USMLE Step 2 Score
Requirement:** 210
Attempts on any step: Must pass on the
first attempt
CS required at time of application: Yes
including ECFMG certificate
USCE Requirement: None
Cut-Off time since graduation: 5 years

Program offers couple match: Yes
Visas Sponsored or accepted: J1 visa

West Virginia University General Surgery Residency Program

Specialty: General Surgery
Program name: West Virginia University Program
Program code: 440-55-21-352
NRMP Code: 1837440P1, 1837440C0
Program type: University-based
State: West Virginia
Address: West Virginia University School of Medicine
              1 Medical Center Dr., Morgantown, WV 26506-9238
Phone: (304) 293-1254
Fax: (304) 293-4711
Percentage of IMGs in the program: 0%
Minimum USMLE Step 1 Score Requirement: No limits set
Minimum USMLE Step 2 Score Requirement: No limits set
Attempts on any step: Must pass on the first attempt
CS required at time of application: Yes including ECFMG certificate
USCE Requirement: None
Cut-Off time since graduation: 2 years

Program offers couple match: Yes
Visas Sponsored or accepted: J1 visa

Marshall University School of Medicine General Surgery Residency Program

Specialty: General Surgery
Program name: Marshall University School of Medicine Program
Program code: 440-55-21-366
NRMP Code: 3066440C0, 3066440P0
Program type: Community-based university affiliated hospital
State: West Virginia
Address: Marshall University School of Medicine
           1600 Medical Center Dr, Huntington, WV 25701
Phone: (304) 691-1282
Percentage of IMGs in the program: 0%
Minimum USMLE Step 1 Score Requirement: 210
Minimum USMLE Step 2 Score Requirement: 210
Attempts on any step: Must pass on the first attempt

Applicants with scores of 230 or above, membership in AOA, etc., may be offered the convenience of a SKYPE interview.
CS required at time of application: Yes including ECFMG certificate
USCE Requirement: 6 months
Cut-Off time since graduation: 2 years
Program offers couple match: Yes
Visas Sponsored or accepted: J1 visa

Wisconsin

Gundersen Lutheran Medical Foundation General Surgery Residency Program

Specialty: General Surgery
Program name: Gundersen Lutheran Medical Foundation Program
Program code: 440-56-12-354
NRMP Code: 1774440C0
Program type: Community-based
State: Wisconsin
Address: Gundersen Medical Foundation
        1836 South Ave, La Crosse, WI 54601-5429
Phone: (608) 775-2431

Fax: (608) 775-7327
Percentage of IMGs in the program: 0%
Minimum USMLE Step 1 Score Requirement: 210
Minimum USMLE Step 2 Score Requirement: 210
Attempts on any step: Must pass on the first attempt
CS required at time of application: Yes including ECFMG certificate
USCE Requirement: 1 year
Cut-Off time since graduation: 2 years
Program offers couple match: Yes
Visas Sponsored or accepted: J1 visa and H1b visa

University of Wisconsin General Surgery Residency Program

Specialty: General Surgery
Program name: University of Wisconsin Program
Program code: 440-56-21-355
NRMP Code: 1779440C0, 1779440P3
Program type: University-based
State: Wisconsin
Address: University of Wisconsin Hospital and Clinics
            600 Highland Ave, Madison, WI 53792-7375

Phone: (608) 263-1377
Fax: (608) 252-0950
Percentage of IMGs in the program: 5%
Minimum USMLE Step 1 Score Requirement:
No limits set
Minimum USMLE Step 2 Score Requirement:
No limits set
Attempts on any step: No limits set
CS required at time of application: Yes
including ECFMG certificate
USCE Requirement: Yes, 1 year
Cut-Off time since graduation: No limits set
Program offers couple match: Yes
Visas Sponsored or accepted: J1 visa

Medical College of Wisconsin Affiliated Hospitals General Surgery Residency Program

Specialty: General Surgery
Program name: Medical College of
Wisconsin Affiliated Hospitals Program
Program code: 440-56-21-357
NRMP Code:
Program type:
State: Wisconsin
Address: Froedtert Memorial Lutheran
Hospital
            9200 W Wisconsin Ave,
Milwaukee, WI 53226

Phone: (414) 805-8632
Fax: (414) 805-5921
Percentage of IMGs in the program: 10%
**Minimum USMLE Step 1 Score
Requirement:** No limits set
**Minimum USMLE Step 2 Score
Requirement:** No limits set
Attempts on any step: Must pass on the
first attempt
CS required at time of application: Yes
including ECFMG certificate
USCE Requirement: None
Cut-Off time since graduation: 3 years
Program offers couple match: Yes
Visas Sponsored or accepted: J1 visa and
H1b visa

Marshfield Clinic-St Joseph's Hospital General Surgery Residency Program

Specialty: General Surgery
Program name: Marshfield Clinic-St Joseph's
Hospital Program
Program code: 440-56-31-356
State: Wisconsin
Address: Marshfield Clinic
          1000 N Oak Ave, Marshfield, WI
54449
Phone: (715) 387-9222

Fax: (715) 221-6687
Percentage of IMGs in the program: 30%
Minimum USMLE Step 1 Score Requirement:
No limits set if you have 1 year USCE otherwise
220 is the minimum
Minimum USMLE Step 2 Score Requirement:
No limits set if you have 1 year USCE otherwise
220 is the minimum
Attempts on any step: Must
CS required at time of application: Yes
including ECFMG certificate
USCE Requirement: None
Cut-Off time since graduation: 3 years
Program offers couple match: Yes
Visas Sponsored or accepted: J1 visa and H1b
visa

I wish you good luck.

Thank you for buying our book.

Please, Please and Please take a minute to review our book on Amazon.

**Match A Doc
Residency Guide**

www.matchadoc.com